A Handbook of
SICK VISITING

by

NORMAN AUTTON

Chaplain: University Hospital of Wales, Cardiff

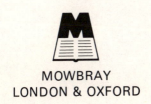

MOWBRAY
LONDON & OXFORD

Copyright © Norman Autton

ISBN 0 264 66779 4

First published 1981
by A. R. Mowbray & Co. Ltd
Saint Thomas House, Becket Street
Oxford, OX1 1SJ

Typeset by Cotswold Typesetting Ltd, Gloucester and Printed in Great
Britain by St Edmundsbury Press, Bury St Edmunds

British Library Cataloguing in Publication Data

Autton, Norman
  A handbook of sick visiting.
  1. Visiting the sick
  I. Title
  362.1   HV696.V/

  ISBN 0-264-66779-4

To Katie, Michael and Mary

Contents

Preface

This handbook of sick visiting has been written not solely for the parish priest but also for the laity so that ministering together as a pastoral team they may form the nucleus of a caring and healing community. To speak of local congregations sharing support, love, prayer and acceptance is to speak of pastoral care. The essential role of the local church is to be a redemptive fellowship, existing not in and for itself but for the health and healing of the total community. Illness should never be seen as an isolated individual event.

The purpose of the following chapters is to provide basic information about some of the main aspects of sick visiting and of the various resources available in both hospital and community. Training, theoretical as well as practical, needs to be well organised and the final section describes in detail various methods which may be employed to help instruct priest and lay-folk. We cannot come to others until we have first come to ourselves. It is essential therefore that we know who we are, what we are, and what we are all about. The search to know ourselves accurately involves effort, a great deal of time, and often much emotional pain. It has been truly said that one of the greatest acts of daring a man can perform is to be himself. Unless we relate to our sick people openly and honestly we shall prompt them to re-echo the words of one patient, who when asked, 'How do you like the people here?', replied, 'There are no people here. There's just doctors, nurses and patients'.

Small groups of trained pastoral teams, with the widest representation in their membership, people of various denominations and different sectors of society, can call forth a unique level of pastoral care. In such a concept of shared leadership in which the christian community moves from the need to receive ministry to a willingness and ability to give ministry, pastor and people become co-partners with mutual roles to play, working together in mission, with a caring responsibility to one another. To become an effective sick visitor is a matter of growth, of being and becoming, of openness to self and to others. Through our caring, our shepherding, our readiness to share the problems and pains of our people, our worth will be measured not so much by the change we may be able to effect in their lives but rather by the level of our involvement and our commitment to them.

In each pastoral encounter we shall have to take the risk of being hurt, of being wounded in the process, as we endeavour to take the pain and the brokenness of the other into our consciousness. In this way we become wounded healers, following in the footsteps of our Lord himself. In the play, *The Angel that troubled the Waters*, by Thornton Wilder, the apparently whole physician is commanded to stand back at the crucial moment, despite his own yearning for wholeness. 'Without your wound where would your power be?' the angel asks. 'In love's service only the wounded soldiers can serve. Draw back'. Such is the challenge that confronts us all.

Finally I wish to express my appreciation to the Revd Canon William Purcell, literary adviser to Messrs Mowbray, for all his help and encouragement, as well as his valuable practical advice and counsel in the preparation of this book. My gratitude is also extended to Mrs Anne Taylor, my secretary, who cheerfully and conscientiously typed the manuscript.

Epiphanytide
1981

Norman Autton

Chapter 1

The Involvement

The very atmosphere of the sickroom at home or in hospital forces us out of a shell of detachment into the arena of life to wrestle with some of the basic issues of life and death—anxiety, fear, loneliness, despair, futility, guilt and estrangement. These feelings comprise the essential components of religious concern. We go out therefore to visit not knowing where we shall be led. Each bedside call is on new territory where we have never been before—to this particular sick person in this particular state. There can be no set procedures, pleasing panaceas or official formulae, for at each sickbed we shall be presented with a unique situation.

The biblical picture of pastoral concern with its challenge and in its comprehensiveness is clearly stipulated in Isaiah 61. 1–3: 'The spirit of the Lord is upon me because the Lord has anointed me; he has sent me to bring good news to the humble, to bind up the broken-hearted, to proclaim liberty to captives and release to those in prison . . . to comfort all who mourn, to give them . . . a garment of splendour for the heavy heart' (NEB). Visiting of the sick is just one of the larger responsibilities of pastoral care, for the scope of pastoral interest is the whole of man's life and in man as a whole.

Some of the unique features of our sick call must first be noted. It will differ from that of the doctor, be he hospital consultant or local practitioner, for obvious reasons. He works as one in complete charge of the sick patient, renders a service to the patient at the patient's request on the basis of expert medical knowledge of the disease or disorder, and his aim is to cure. The sick visitor, be he priest or layman, comes, whether or not at the patient's request, without any specialised knowledge of the disorder. He stands by and ministers not so much to cure as to care, to share the joy or sorrow, to reveal Christ in all circumstances. It is true that some of the same difficulties and concerns will often face both ministries but differentiation of functions will not mean separation or isolation.

Our pastoral care will also differ in certain respects from that of the social worker. Both will impinge much on the ministries of the other but here again there are differences. Usually the social worker has been directed to the patient via the doctor and is concerned primarily with the here and now, for case-work concentrates on helping people cope with a specific problem. The visit of the priest or minister attempts to help the sick deal with the whole of life, its meaning and purpose. He will work at once in the sphere of the temporal and the eternal.

One of the finest of all instruments in sick-visiting is that of personality. In a sense the visitor or counsellor himself is the most important part of the 'good news' he has come to bring. Everything will depend upon the relationships of person to person in the interactive fellowship of a loving community. Our personal attitudes and influences are among our greatest resources, for we can offer our sick nothing better than creative meaningful relationships. This involves making ourselves vulnerable to each other, being attentive and alert to God and to others. We have to be the kind of person who helps others find their own true relationship to God, so that they may become whatever in the grace of God they can become.

Sick-visiting is a very costly experience. 'Why do you keep what we need most from us—yourself?' asked one patient. 'Don't you know that if you don't give us something of yourself as a person you can't mean anything to us at all!' There can be no understanding of others unless we ourselves are prepared and able to reveal ourselves. We shall find that generally speaking the sick will wait for us to reveal ourselves, and their own self-revelation will be governed by the quality of what we reveal about ourselves. Only then are we able to centre our attention and care on the individual sick person before us and discover the deeper meaning of our life in mutual association together. Jesus attracted and helped people through his love and affection for them. We shall do well to try and follow his example.

Those who are ill are often temporarily insecure and self-conscious. It is important therefore that everything should be done to make them feel at ease in our presence. One of the best ways of achieving this will be to be at ease ourselves. Those first few moments at the bedside are of vital importance, for it is in this initial stage that the visit will prove effective or otherwise. We follow the clues of what we see and hear, being quick to observe signs, postures, motions, expressions. We ask ourselves questions. 'What does God require of me at this bedside?' 'What is he showing me?' 'What, if anything, does he want me to do or to say?' 'How am I going to establish a relationship with this sick person which he may use for the person's personal and spiritual growth?'

One of our most important roles at this stage will be to understand. When the sick person realises we understand he derives the greatest comfort from our presence. It is the agonising feeling of aloneness or of being misunderstood which saps the strength and weakens the will. Visiting another in sickness is first and foremost an exercise in understanding, in assessment of need, and in desire and effort to meet that need. We have to create an atmosphere of warm receptiveness, of acceptance, of confidence and trust, so that conversation on a deep and personal level can flow freely and fully.

We have as great a need to understand the sick person

before us and to know how to deal with his fears, anxieties, and difficulties, as a physician has to understand the human body and treat its disorders. Like the doctor we too have to learn to acquire the art of 'diagnosis'. Before we can visit effectively we must be able to grasp things as they really are, to acquire a discerning knowledge and understanding of human ills and the needs and conditions of sick people. In its original derivation the word 'diagnosis' means 'to know through and through'. To minister adequately we have to try to know fully the persons whom we are visiting, in all their joys and sorrows, in all their 'ups and downs'. As Matthew Arnold said of Goethe:

He took the suffering human race;
He read each wound, each weakness clear;
And stuck his finger on the place
And said, Thou ailest here, and here.

Yet all must be done in a spirit of true compassion, humility and love. We shall so direct the conversation that the patient may achieve insight through the talking out of his fears and anxieties, rather than that he passively accept or reject a 'diagnosis' authoritatively imposed upon him. We shall do well to pray with St Paul that 'our love may grow ever richer and richer in knowledge and insight of every kind, and may thus bring us *the gift of true discrimination*'. (Philippians 1.9 NEB). A sick person will never be helped if he expects one thing and is given another; if he asks for 'bread' and is given a 'stone' (Matthew 7.9). Such a ministry makes great demands upon us and calls for the utmost skill, sensitivity, diligence and careful consideration of the appropriate aspect of our pastoral care.

What are some of the main phases of our relationship with the sick whom we visit at home or in hospital? First will come the *orientation* phase. When we arrive at the bedside we pay careful attention to what patients say because it is then that they outline the area with which at that moment they are particularly concerned. Here is set the model for the later phases. We shall introduce ourselves, telling patients our name and also get to know theirs, for identity is most important. Within this given framework patients are now free to proceed at their own pace, in their own way, and in the direction of their own personal choice. They may then be encouraged to talk about themselves, their present concerns and their current experiences.

In this initial stage of our visit our manner, approach and poise should be as matter-of-fact and relaxed as possible. As yet we do not really know the sick person neither does he know us. We express some individuality in the tone of voice we use, the choice of words we make, and the kind of attention we give. The patients' contributions at this early stage may be confused, and their statements unrelated, as a result of pain or anxiety. If however we let ourselves hear what they say, no matter how disjointed their words may seem, and how they say them, we shall soon get an idea of the key concepts or ideas which underlie these statements and which bind them into shape. We shall then be aware of three kinds of underlying key ideas or themes:— the *content* theme, the *mood* theme and the theme of *interaction*. While we listen to the theme underlying the *what* of patients' communications we also listen to *how* they get it across. Do they feel frightened?—the mood may be fear or anxiety. Do they seem sorry for themselves?—the theme or key idea may be self-pity or mere depression. Do they seem defiant?—it may be that the mood is anger and frustration. As they continue to talk we shall either be confirmed in our original impressions or we shall have to revise our assumption. But the chances are that if we have really listened to what patients say and how they come across we shall not be very far wrong in picking up these key themes. We must guard against attempting to find causes of problems prematurely, for the cause will become apparent only after all the facts are in. By listening for the cause of the problem we may well miss hearing what patients are trying to communicate.

We shall note in what way we are received by the sick

whom we visit. Their reaction and behaviour towards us, and equally important our response to them, will constitute the interaction theme. It is important therefore that during the orientation phase we be not mere passive listeners but that we listen in such a way as to help patients give vent to their areas of concern.

The second phase will be the *working* one. How long the orientation phase takes and at what point this second phase begins will vary tremendously with each particular patient; more often than not it will be gradual, for it rarely happens all at once. If patients are very anxious or depressed the relationship may never progress beyond the initial phase. What marks out this working phase of our visit? Generally speaking it is during this time that patients fill in the picture which they have outlined during the orientation phase and they begin to come to grips with their experience. We are now in a position to help patients cope with the experiences that confront them, for example, by listening, responding, or through prayer, bible-reading and sacrament.

How do we recognise that patients have reached this working phase? A marked sign is that they will be expecting our visit, and are waiting and ready to talk, usually about topics referred to in the orientation period. Perhaps they will need some further questions to help them enlarge upon their descriptions so that a more complete picture can emerge. This is most important, for if no help is forthcoming from ourselves patients may tend to go over the same story in the same way as before, without gaining much relief from it, or any deeper understanding.

As this working phase progresses and after patients have given us a rather full description of the specific areas with which they are at present concerned, we shall assist them further to abstract the themes most significant for their situations and look at the component parts of each theme. Through patience and encouragement we hope to sustain them as they are led to new insights into their present predicaments. More often than not we shall have very little time or opportunity to work through the entire process. This does not mean, however, that we should be disappointed or attempt to take shortcuts to reach final goals. It takes time for a building to be erected and sometimes the process may have to be halted for a while. The main thought is that the foundations laid are solid and secure.

Finally there will be the *closing* phase. Whenever possible the termination phase should be built into the relationship from the very first meeting or visit. If the patient is in hospital and the discharge date is at all foreseeable then the fact should be kept in mind and openly discussed during the visits. In this way patients have opportunity to gauge how much they may want to share with us in the time allotted. Also we shall have to decide how far we can possibly go and what will have to be referred.

Words are among the most sensitive instruments of precision in a sickroom, for with them the most delicate operations will have to be performed. Intonations and reflections of voice give expression that can enrich the meaning of the words. The right word at the right time can be a means of grace. We may talk too much but never too well. We must needs learn to understand the language by which persons, including ourselves, not only reveal but conceal themselves. Words become shallow and hollow when they bear little relevance to the situation at hand. Our constant plea will be: 'Pray for me that I may be granted the right words when I open my mouth. . .' (Ephesians 6.19 NEB). Speech reveals the speaker. 'The way you speak gives you away'. (Matthew 26.73 Good News Bible). When our words express an openness of ourselves speech becomes sharing. 'Let your conversation be always gracious, and never insipid', advised St Paul. (Colossians 4.6 NEB) 'Study how best to talk with each person you meet'. Such speech will neither manipulate nor control but will aim at self-giving, at liberating, at not only helping but healing. Words must be chosen wisely and discretely and should be kept as simple as possible. Ideas too should be clear and repeated and rephrased whenever necessary. It is when we speak and act from the depths of our total self that we become creative channels between the sick and ourselves. True dialogue has been defined as 'that interaction between persons in which one of them seeks to give himself as he is to the other, and seeks also to know the other as the other is'.

Thoughtless words can be damaging. Considered words, precisely tailored to anticipate anxiety or fear, can be healing. We shall use words not merely for something to say but out of respect for, and interest in, the patient. Clear and simple speech will prove the best method of verbal communication. Where there is no real dialogue we become 'as strangers talking to strangers about something they did not want to hear about', for there can be no meaningful relationship where there is no understanding of what we say at the bedside. As well as an aid to communication language can sometimes be a barrier. 'I know you think you understand what you think I said. But I am sure you realise that what you heard is what I meant'. (Anon)

One of the most popular 'games people play' at the bedsides of the sick is that of firing questions. It takes time to get to know a patient and it is always best that each unfolds himself to the other at his own pace. So often we prod with questions, not knowing what to say to the stranger in the bed. In our anxiety and insecurity we try and keep the conversation going with a barrage of questions; 'Where are you from? Have you been in long? Do you have any visitors? Have you had your operation yet?'. Do we really get to know sick people in this way? Many a bedside conversation develops into a sort of versicle and response. The sick answer our questions as laconically as they can but they must often wish that we would stop cross-questioning them so that they can really concentrate on what is bothering them and put it into words. Too frequent questioning implies that we stand opposite, or over and against, rather than alongside the patient, so eager are we to direct the conversation and hold the reins. We shall find that questions, if they have to be asked, are far more profitable towards the end of the visit when we are beginning to know each other and learn what each is about.

Where questions are asked they have to be handled skilfully, avoiding those which merely evoke a 'yes' or a 'no'. What a scalpel is to a surgeon so is a question to the sick-visitor, and often quite as dangerous a tool. The surgeon knows what to cut and what not to cut—so too should the good sick visitor. The art is to know what questions to ask and when and how probing and searching they should be. If we do not ask the right questions we shall not get the right answers. When too many questions are asked we deny the sick the opportunity of expressing their concerns and ourselves the chance of hearing how they explain them. Some questions are often necessary during a pastoral call but they should be spaced out during the visit and phrased in as neutral and open-ended a way as possible.

Those who visit the sick should resist all temptation to moralise, dogmatise, preach or admonish. Moralising means standing in opposition to the sick person and losing all contact of togetherness. The patient will soon feel misunderstood and set aside by such responses as 'you must', or 'you mustn't', 'you should' or 'you shouldn't'. To sermonise is to take unfair advantage of the 'captive' patient and stand over and above the bedridden victim.

Doctrinal 'capsules' are to be handed out with great caution in the sick room. To generalise is to disturb the flow of feelings and emotions of the patient. Another common but unfortunate habit is to discuss and describe in gruesome detail one's own complaints or operations; a kind of 'pathological conference', or a boring and long drawn-out 'organ recital'. Neither is it helpful to point out other patients in the hospital ward who might be in much worse condition in an attempt to reassure. The average patient derives but little comfort and consolation from a knowledge of other people's ills!

Speaking and hearing are a total process. As we hear so we

speak. The rhythm of listening and speaking has been likened to an alternative current in which listening intervenes between speaking and doing to inform and guide all we do. The good sick visitor will listen rather than talk, understand than judge, wait patiently than hurry, and give information rather than advice. He will listen with his eyes and heart as well as his ears. In *Staircase for Silence*, Alan Ecclestone states that 'it has been said with justice that it is not so much the gift of tongues that we now need as the gift of ears, not so much the proclamation of our beliefs as the willingness to listen to the ways in which we ourselves are being addressed, not so much the assertion of our knowledge but the silent admission that we are ready to learn . . .' (p. 41). 'A new vision of hell is conjured up as perceiving a state where no one ceases to talk and no one listens'. (p 48). Listening, that 'certain, difficult concentration' (Simone Weil), is an art that all sick visitors have to cultivate. We have to listen to the meaning of words and to the whole personality of the patient. How true it is that:

> Words are like leaves, and where they most abound
> Much fruit of sense beneath is rarely found. (Pope)

Words should always be weighed not counted.

Listening is neither easy nor simple. To listen is to concentrate, to accept fully the speaker, to be unfailingly honest and transparently real. It is something far more profound than merely keeping quiet. Intelligent listening means that we as visitors are not only listening but also understanding, giving our full attention not only to what is being said but also to what is being felt. True listening is both active and creative, not only in the sense that we must be actively concentrating, but also that we have in listening a most effective way of talking and of communicating attitudes which are so important and significant. The listening ear is of no less importance than the speaking mouth, for listening must come first if we are to speak meaningfully. The vague stare, or mechanical nod or the blank smile is not to be mistaken for listening. We have to catch every implication and shade of meaning, note every gesture and postural expression, follow each clue and relate fragments and hints into larger patterns of understanding. We have to listen to questions rather than search for answers. Often we shall find, much to our surprise, that our sick people are helped and cheered, not by anything we say or do, but by our silent and sustaining interest which has led them to discover that which they had not found before. Our listening seems to give them new power to meet and answer questions aroused by their predicament, and to draw them out to say more than they started to say, to answer themselves better than we could answer for them. Through the speaking and the listening something happens to the both of us. Each of us is recreated. A new reality seems to spring up between us and both of us are changed.

'Healers are hosts who patiently and carefully listen to the story of the suffering strangers,' writes Henri Nouwen. 'Patients are guests who rediscover their selves by telling their story to the one who offers them a place to stay. In the telling of their stories, strangers befriend not only their host but also their own past. So healing is the receiving and full understanding of the story so that strangers can recognise in the eyes of their host their own unique way that leads them to the present and suggests the direction in which to go'.[1] We have to bear in mind that we shall not be able to listen to others more deeply than we have listened to ourselves; we shall not be able to speak to the depths of our sick people until we have learned to listen to our own deeper feelings and meanings.

We can listen only if we have the gift of quietness. Busyness is the frantic mood of the unfulfilled life to which far too many of us fall prey. Quietness is not merely the absence of noise, but a quality of spirit that suggests a perfect union with God. It partakes of a pervading peace which upholds life in a

[1] *Reaching Out* (Fontana) 1980. p. 89.

sufficient strength to meet and accept whatever may come. Its message comes not in wind, earthquake or fire but in the still small voice of calm. Quietness is contagious and it may be one of the most precious gifts we can bring to the sickroom. If we are to be welcomed we have to be quiet men and women. 'Study to be quiet', the writer of I Thessalonians 4.11 tells us. In the NEB it is translated: 'Let it be your ambition to keep calm.' No sick person will unfold his worries and concerns to us if we are constantly looking at our watch, stressing how very busy we are, or muttering, 'Isn't life hectic'.

Through our listening and our quietness we are able to penetrate the other's feelings comprehendingly and so establish a spirit of empathy and acceptance. Empathy has been defined as 'your pain in my heart'. It is that state of identification of personalities in which one person so feels himself into the other as temporarily to lose his own identity. It sees a sick person not primarily as 'someone to be helped' but rather a friend to be loved. It is in this mysterious process that understanding, influence and other significant relationships take place. It was Adler who once stated that 'it is impossible to understand another individual if it is impossible at the same time to identify one's self with him'. Empathy is akin to sympathy yet distinct from it. Empathy says, 'I know how you feel'; sympathy says, 'I feel as you do'. Empathy is often the more therapeutic of the two for it is objective and includes all that is of value in sympathy.

It has been said that while words are like the lines of a painting, non-verbal action fills out the picture with colour and shade. The facial expressions, sighs and gestures of the sick can convey far more significant information than anything which can be expressed in words, and as visitors we should always be on the alert, ready to read and interpret such body-language. Our eyes will watch for tell-tale signs of distress, fear, sadness, anger, the nervous laugh and the forced cheerfulness. A smile, a frown, a raised eyebrow, eyes that will not meet ours, are all conveying emotional states.

'When the eyes say one thing, and the tongue another', said Emerson, 'a practised man relies on the language of the first'. The face is a most revealing communicator; it provides us with non-verbal feed-back from others as we speak to them. 'There are mystically in our faces certain characters which carry in them the motto of our souls, wherein he that cannot read ABC may read our natures', wrote Sir Thomas Browne in his *Religio Medici* (1642).

Hands too are important instruments for expressing non-verbal communication. Frequently hand-gestures accompany and reinforce speech. The nervous patient will clutch or crinkle bed-clothes, the fearful and agitated wipe perspiring hands. Hands held out to touch those of another will speak of loneliness, isolation, despair, or will seek for relief in pain or discomfort. Immeasurable support and comfort are given to sick people by taking their hand, or placing one's arm around them in times of depression or stress. The importance of touch in nursing has been described in the following statement by S. Roberts in *Behavioural concepts and the critically ill patient* (Prentice-Hall, New Jersey, 1976). 'Sometimes machines make data collection too easy. The nurse may begin to rely on the machines for data instead of her own eyes and judgement. Reliance on machines diminishes the amount of sensory input from touch. When the nurse limits her touching to the patient's equipment, the patient experiences emotional deprivation'. A touch of a hand or the clasp of a palm can express more love and compassion than can ever be given verbally. Physical touch should always be used spontaneously, never forced or calculated.

In our eagerness to express pity and sympathy we can very readily give way to reassurances and 'silver-lining' approaches—'Don't worry, you'll probably feel much better tomorrow'. 'You must look on the bright side'. 'Everything's going to be all right'. Clichés are marks of slipshod thinking and they are far too common in sick-visiting. Reassurance, while not without value in some circumstances, is less effective than the kind of calm, quiet acceptance that enables the sick person to gain intrinsic confidence in himself. Reassurance from someone else can prove superficial and is often resented, for the sick are being told that they need not feel the way they are actually feeling. Consequently they feel they are not being taken seriously. We shall soon find that reassurances do not normally reassure but serve rather to increase anxiety in the mind of the patient. We have not far to look to discover the reason why—our need to reassure others grows out of our own anxieties, for the persons we are really trying to reassure are ourselves!

Reassurance can often be unrealistic and tend only to repress feelings and problems which need to be expressed, accepted and understood. Superficial assurance disrupts rather than develops our relationship with those which we visit. Genuine affection for sick people leads us to accept them as they are. The role of the visitor is to mirror attitudes and feelings which at that moment are contained in the patient's expressions, rather than to try to bring up topics which he himself feels are significant and interesting. It is the patient who is the expert on his particular concerns and he should be left to state them *as* he wishes and *when* he wishes. We can be together at the bedside and yet not meet as person to person.

Interest and caring will prove far more important that the acquisition of 'techniques'. By way of warning we can recall the story of the famous centipede which got on very well until it began to think of how it managed to get its feet forward in the correct order and consequently came to a full stop. In like manner technique may lead to impotence. If we become tied and bound to technical 'know-hows' we shall no longer be listening to what our patient is saying but to what we can do with what he is saying. We cannot hear when we are absorbed in our own anticipations and expectations.

All information about those whom we visit either in hospital or at home must be kept in the strictest confidence. So easily can we divulge to others what is confidential material and Mr X's medical diagnosis and prognosis can soon become common knowledge throughout the parish. We must always hold sacred what is told us in private. Neither will the experienced visitor ask the patient about his particular complaint. His illness is the sick person's personal and private concern and if he wishes the visitor to know he will tell him himself without being faced with embarrassing questions. Neither will we ask the nursing staff about medical details or casenote minuting regarding patients. It is to be hoped that through good inter-personal relationships sufficient information will be forthcoming whereby our visit may be made as fruitful and profitable as possible. The privacy of each individual patient in hospital has to be strictly observed. Patients form part of a large 'captive' audience and although we shall endeavour to make ourselves available and accessible to all we shall need to respect the personal privacy of each.

In hospital the sick-visitor will often be meeting patients who do not specifically call themselves 'christians', or who are indifferent to spiritual things. If he is prepared to chat in a friendly way and express concern and interest in them as persons he will rarely meet with any resentment or aloofness. He will minister to them as person-to-person, as friend-to-friend. Where suspicion or misunderstanding does exist it may soon be overcome by a spirit of respect and companionship. Religious debates or arguments are completely out of place at the bedsides of the sick.

Finally we have to realise we are members of a team and our ministry will only be effective in so far as we are willing and able to co-ordinate our own work with that of others who are serving the sick in hospital or in community. It is only by such mutual confidence that the total care of the patient will be achieved. We shall try to get to know as many staff members as possible, for doctors, ward-sisters/charge-nurses, nursing officers and social workers will be our constant guides within the hospital. In the community we must needs liaise closely with general practitioners, community nurses, health visitors and social workers. Whether they are aware of it or not they are all members of the-church-in-hospital/community fulfilling the redemptive work of Christ in a sick world. Many may be shy or reticent about claiming any christian allegiance, yet their religious anonymity may sometimes open a way to trust and confidence among their patients where our official 'church image' may inhibit or constrain.

The last word about the sick person and his treatment will always be the prerogative of the doctor and the members of his team, but we shall have much to contribute to the total concern of the patient if we have been conscientious in our visiting, in our co-operation with hospital or community resources, in our understanding of certain features of the illness, and in our awareness of the patient's emotional and spiritual reactions. Where such a working relationship exists only rarely will any major problems arise from our work together. Each of us will be ready to listen to and learn from the other and work alongside the other for the patient's health, environment, and relationships. If this be so the whole climate of healing in hospital and home will thereby be enhanced.

Thus far we have been discussing our function and role as sick-visitors and how best we can play our part in meeting the needs of the sick. It is equally important that we understand what it means to be a patient and so in the next chapter we take note of some of the emotional and psychological reactions of 'being sick'.

Chapter 2

The Patient

When a person is sick the outer world seems to recede in importance as he is absorbed into a new inner strange personal land of mystery, lostness, isolation and dependence. The horizon appears to shrink and the patient creates a world of his own, an inner world, all of whose occupants are sick. He becomes dependent upon all about him as he finds himself 'under doctor's orders'. 'The simple everyday rules that govern the way we act are changed for the sick. Though their world and ours look the same, sound the same, are the same, the rules are different, as in a science fiction story in which an alien from another planet invades an earthman's body and takes over. Nobody can tell because to all appearances the earthling is still the same, and thereby hangs the danger'.[1]

A sick person is a frightened person. The popular concept still permeates the thinking of many when admission to hospital is mentioned—'it must be something serious'. A mental picture of the hospital as a fearsome, even if wondrous, place grows easily. The larger the hospital and the further distance it is from the home area the more awesome and frightening it appears to be. Fears of suffering and death, an inability to deal with the demands of everyday living, separation from family and friends and disruption of the

[1] *The Healer's Art*, Eric J. Cassell, Penguin Books, 1978. p. 23.

normal pattern of life confront and torment the mind. The sick person is now part of a new and frightening world—'the world of the sick', and is obliged to assume the 'sick role', with its loss of customary rights, privileges and satisfactions. The most common stresses encountered in illness are fear and anxiety, increased irritability, unhappiness, loss of interest in the outside world, and preoccupation with bodily processes. The uncertainty of not knowing what is going to happen causes much anxiety and apprehension. Hospitalisation enforces separation and strangeness.

There are certain characteristic phases to be found in all illness. First of all there is the *transition* period from health to sickness, which may be either sudden or gradual. It is a time which is often characterised by fear and anxiety either at an overt and conscious level or at a deeper subconscious level which inhibits open verbal expression. Next comes the *treatment* phase with its marked dependency patterns. Symptoms have now to be faced and dealt with, a diagnosis to be made. High levels of anxiety are normally experienced by those who have to undergo surgical operations or diagnostic procedures, for there can be no such thing as 'a minor operation' for those concerned. Individual emotional traits will obviously affect how various people react to sickness and how they respond to particular events while in hospital or at home. Finally there follows the period of *convalescence*, often the most difficult phase of all and a largely neglected sphere of pastoral care. Transition has now to be made from a temporary dependency role to assuming once again the responsibilities of everyday life and work.

Reactions to 'being a patient' will obviously vary from individual to individual, but there are common implications to which all sick people react. If in hospital the patient will be in unfamiliar surroundings, be subject to unaccustomed routines and restrictions, and may well suffer lack of privacy. He will be confronted by strange faces, and exposed to fears of the unknown. As he becomes more and more oriented to hospital life 'the strange white world' gradually becomes 'his world', and all who enter from the 'outside,' including his own familiar kith and kin, become visitors from some 'distant world'. The focus of his attention begins to shift and he asks such questions as, 'How long will I have to be in? What will be the eventual outcome of my illness? Will I have to undergo surgery? What about my future employment, my family, etc.?' The presence of other patients about him will either have a supportive and comforting effect on him or will distress and embarrass him. He now has to learn to adjust, to become accustomed to life in hospital and become part of it. The unfamiliar can often be bewildering and frightening for he is no longer in control of the situation; others are now in charge. His normal everyday time-table has had to be abandoned. He is told when to eat meals, when to go to bed, and when to get up.[1] He is subjected to various tests, medical procedures and examinations, many of which are unpleasant and whose purposes are not always explained to him. The extent to which he becomes satisfied with what information he receives is normally related to how much he really wants to know.

Having submitted to such rituals he now has to await results and can only hope they will be favourable. Everyone about him seems particularly busy whilst he is in enforced idleness. Little wonder therefore that there is so much emotional regression, for such dependence has a marked effect upon sick people. All illness has a tendency to force one to give up some of the prerogatives associated with maturity. A patient is admitted to a protective environment, freed from responsibility, and forced to adopt an entirely passive and submissive attitude. The very derivation of the word 'patient' is interesting and intriguing—'one who waits or one who suffers or endures'. He is therefore expected to conform and 'put up with things'; to be obedient, passive, accepting rather than an intelligent, co-operative person, thinking and acting spontaneously. Consequently he searches for two comforting and consoling symbols and becomes emotionally dependent

[1] Vide Appendix 3.

upon the strong and capable 'father' figure (doctor) and the understanding, sympathetic and tender 'mother' (nurse).

The longer a person remains in hospital the more attention he concentrates on self. He will normally bring to his illness similar patterns of behaviour and some of the same reactions that characterised his life prior to the onset of his admission when in good health, although his particular illness may bring these more significantly to the forefront.

Psychological and emotional concepts will depend a great deal on the *age* of the sick person. Young children separated from mother and familiar home surroundings will often experience feelings of abandonment and desolation. Adults will vary considerably in their reactions. The majority seem to 'take it all in their stride', with a philosophical outlook of 'it's just one of those things'! There will be others, particularly adult males, who will be inclined to suppress their emotions. The *illness* of the patient will have a major effect on his emotional outlook. A short stay, either in hospital or at home, with a minor complaint will have little effect upon him, but if faced with a chronic illness he can very readily give way to feelings of rejection, anger and frustration. Major surgery will very naturally arouse haunting fears and anxieties. Another deciding factor is the *personality* of the patient. The majority of well adjusted persons will adapt quite adequately and are able to work satisfactorily through periods of anxiety and depression. Some types of personality will *revel* in the companionship of other patients and become the life and soul of the ward; others will *rebel* and dread every moment of their experience. *Social circumstances* will also influence the reactions of a patient to his new surroundings in hospital. Interpersonal relationships within the family will colour his response. The lonely and those with few friends will have ambivalent feelings, for they look forward to being fit and well again but know they will miss on discharge the friendship and camaraderie of a hospital ward. Problems of having to leave a young family or aged parents at home may create guilt feelings as well as anxiety in many a patient.

Among the most crucial factors that influence the way a patient is likely to perceive, interpret and respond to what is happening to him in sickness are his condition and what his condition means to him. All these emotions have to be borne in mind by the sick-visitor, for the physical organ effected may be the least important factor in the illness of the patient. An experienced visitor views illness as a manifestation of the whole person, and avoids the tendency to see only the patient's sickness and not the 'person' who is sick. He will ask himself not so much, 'what sort of illness has this person?' but rather, 'what sort of person has this illness?' Such a concept will have many implications and open ways to new understandings of illness and health.

Illness is a particularly severe form of psychological stress, and its most common responses are anxiety, guilt, shame, helplessness, which will naturally vary in quality, duration and intensity. There are feelings not only of deprivation, the patient having been stripped of privacy, home-life, and work, but also of isolation and loss of identity. The fact of pain brings to mind the possibility of death, and such contemplation tends to populate the inner consciousness of the physically ill patient. He may not be seriously ill but his very incapacity is a reminder to him of his finitude, the shortness of life and the certainty of its end. In the minds of many a patient such thoughts take on the character of an apprehensiveness, vague and undefined.

Feelings of anxiety and depression usually last for a few days after a patient's admission to hospital but adjustment is soon made when friendships are established and he becomes more and more familiar with various procedures and with other people in the ward. Sickness is a great leveller and is no respecter of persons. In pyjamas all men are equal. Whatever his station or status a sick person is levelled in a setting provided for and sustained by others: the staff.

There are innumerable ways in which the condition of the patient and his experience can interact and influence one another, and it is well for the sick visitor to be made aware of them. Five broad categories may profitably be described. The patient can be overwhelmed by his condition; he can protect himself from conscious awareness of it by irrational mechanisms of escape; although fully aware of his condition he may appear to be unable or unwilling to accept it; he can use his condition for ulterior purposes, and finally, he can accept his condition. We now look at each category in turn.

A patient who has suffered a stroke, for example, or been severely handicapped as a result of an accident, often finds his condition so overwhelming to him that he feels it impossible to defend himself against its impact. Such a reaction may not be entirely due to the current effect of his incapacity but as to what he anticipates its effects to be in the not-too-distant future. He also becomes acutely depressed by the implication of his condition for his view of himself. He feels he can never be the same again, for he now lacks virility and his manhood has been impaired. A woman having undergone an operation for mastectomy may become completely shattered by having to acknowledge the fact that she now has a mutilated figure and has lost a vital part of her womanhood. Such a patient often feels less and less able to cope with her condition. Given time, however, it is to be hoped that patients we have been describing will no longer be victims of their condition and completely at its mercy, but will align themselves to those inner and outer forces that have tried to liberate them from its hold.

Another group of patients may well express their feelings of subjection in an entirely different form, giving up all hope of gaining any satisfaction from life even though they may not be seriously incapacitated as a result of their illness. They seem to be utilising to their best advantage the positive opportunities open to them. They lose interest and adopt an entirely pessimistic outlook on life. They cannot or do not want to make an effort to get well again, and give way to resignation. It takes time for patients suffering from cancer, for example, or those whose self-image is threatened, to take in what has happened to them and to re-align themselves with it.

Many patients deny the existence of their condition, in spite of objective evidence to the contrary. They protect themselves from conscious awareness of their condition by irrational mechanisms of escape. It will not do to reason with them for if they could listen to reason they would not have to act in the way they do. They are not able to confront their condition with a conscious mind, and so cannot be held responsible or blamed for this defence behaviour. Patients in this category may well be convinced that there is nothing seriously wrong with them. They will tell you they are only in hospital for 'tests' or 'observation', and will 'probably be home again in a few days'. All the other patients in the ward may have cancer but they are 'only in for back pain'. Slowly perhaps the meaning of what this is all about may well penetrate into their awareness. The process should not be hurried for otherwise they will become very frightened and have to retreat from it.

There will be a number of patients who although fully aware of their conditions are either unable or unwilling to accept them. As a result of this non-acceptance many will have delayed seeing their doctor and seeking medical aid. When they are eventually admitted to hospital their condition has deteriorated, and fear of finding out the truth may change a normally cheerful and outgoing disposition into a depressed, moody and withdrawn personality. Sometimes patients will try to undo what has happened by dwelling on what would have occurred if they or someone else had taken a different course of action at a certain time. This can be termed the 'if only . . .' approach—'If only I had gone by bus and not by car the accident would never have happened'. 'If only I had gone to see the doctor as soon as I had the pain'. 'If only I had given up smoking years ago'. The sick-visitor may well meet patients who feel they have been victimised or singled out. Why should this illness have smitten them, of all people? How very unfair life can be! They resent the fact that sickness should have befallen them.

Some people will take advantage and use their condition

for ulterior purposes. Sickness may well be for them an occasion of abdicating responsibilities, or having a rest, extra comfort and attention. Illness can become a 'secondary gain' in order to avoid solving problems. While out of circulation for a while, patients find that the problem resolves itself. They may well resort to becoming ill whenever they do not know how to cope with a situation or whenever communication with others becomes stressful or strained. There are patients who seem to gain a degree of personal prestige for themselves in being proud of their hospital admissions and series of operations. They apparently possess little else in life than their ailments and the need to have these attended to medically or surgically. They seem proud to exhibit their scars and are quite oblivious to what distress their illnesses cause to their families.

Fortunately the majority of patients seem to accept their condition and are able to make the best of their lives in spite of their sickness without unduly complaining about it, without needing to resent it, and without capitalising on it. This however does not happen spontaneously. Many patients, even those who eventually reach this stage of acceptance, have probably had to struggle through a number of the other phases described above. Again the stage of acceptance is not necessarily a static one. There may be times during spasms of acute pain or moods of acute depression when they may well have to revert, for the time being at least, to less mature ways of coping with their condition.

Sickness affords an opportunity for a patient to think. Whether ill at home or in hospital his day is long and time hangs heavily. It is inevitable that at intermittent periods throughout his sickness there be recollection and reflection. Perhaps for the first time in his life he now has time to concentrate his thoughts on his own and other's experience. 'This illness is certainly making me think', is a remark often heard at the bedside. There can be little escape from his examining himself, his relationships, his world, and the ground and source of life itself.

Illness confronts us with an experience of brokenness, of dis-ease, for the wholeness of life has been disrupted. Life is temporarily estranged and separated from its dynamic wholeness. A sick person inevitably feels frustrated not only as a result of his physical disability but also on an emotional level as he finds his personal relationships becoming more and more distorted. Infusing both the physical and the mental is the dimension of the spiritual in which the patient can lack adequate meaning for life. The interpenetration of a sick body, mind and spirit inhibits him from fully relating to himself, to others and to God, the ground and source of life.

Self-estrangement, the turning in against oneself, is often one of the inevitable symptoms of being sick. Indeed a modern psychiatrist can speak of 'man against himself'. A schism develops between our true essential selves and our apparent existential selves. 'Two souls alas dwell in my breast apart', cried Faust. Because we are not ourselves in sickness we can often be at war with ourselves.

Separation from others, isolation, fear, the very busyness of all about, serve only to devaluate the patient and deepen his sense of loneliness. In the hospital situation inner feelings of unworthiness and apartness are thrust to the fore. He may be on a ward alongside a dozen other patients yet what he is concerned about is his own state, his own pain and his own healing. 'We are never so aware of our separate individuality as when we suffer', writes H. A. Williams. 'Suffering always involves an aloneness, a being cut off from others. Here we are with our pain—physical or mental— and for the rest of the world it is business as usual ... Suffering excludes us from life in the very act of draining it from us.'[1]

In sickness, as we have already noted, there is a constant search for meaning. 'Why has this happened to me?' 'What is the sense of it all?' 'What have I done to deserve this?' As well as separation from self and from others there is also separation from the very reality that overcomes futility and

[1] *True Resurrection*, Mitchell Beazley, 1972. p. 133

despair, making life meaningful and worthwhile—God himself.

The dominant concern of the sick visitor is therefore that of reconciliation, to help bind up the brokenness that man might be whole again with a proper functioning of all his physical, emotional and spiritual resources. He must needs bring those who feel cut off to a sense of meaning and purpose in life, to a realisation that their lives are rooted and grounded in a God who cares for, accepts and encourages them in their struggles for life. He will attempt to bring to light some of their inner destructive emotions, for while there are discordant elements within they will always be at war with themselves. He will strive to create a warm, understanding, accepting relationship at the bedside, for in a free atmosphere the sick will be more ready to express what they feel. He will make every effort to bridge the isolation and loneliness which illness brings in its train. What is important here is not so much what the priest will say or do but what is conveyed by his very presence at the bedside; the being and the being with, the reality of genuine love, concern and care. He will not be able to accomplish this on his own of course and will need the help of a supportive and caring community. Members of the congregation and small groups of trained laity will be alongside him to foster good relationships, to combat loneliness and brokenness so rife in almost every form of sickness. Together they will add the intangible and unexpendable element—people who care about people.

No sick patient should be seen or ministered to 'in vacuo', as an isolated individual. As a pebble thrown into a pond so his illness creates ever expanding circles, affecting his family, relatives and friends. He should therefore always be seen as an integral part of his family and a member of the community in which he lives. The individual is part of the family, and the family a part of the individual. 'When one of us is sick, we're all pretty sick', remarked one patient as he thought of himself and his family. As with individuals so with families there can be no generalisation of reaction or response for each will be affected in different ways. Families after all are composed of individuals. A great deal will depend upon inter-personal relationships within the family group, and on the diagnosis and prognosis of the illness. Family attitudes will vary with the different stages of the illness, whether the family member is in hospital or at home, and whether the patient is the father or mother of the family. If the person is sick at home the minutiae of the everyday household routine may well be disrupted and so deprive young children of the care and attention they need and expect. Their interests may now be given or relegated to a secondary position. Sacrifices may have to be made which will create emotional strain and stress for all concerned. Should the sick member be seen as no more than a passive onlooker in the home, its running and organisation, he can easily become more and more aware of his helplessness and inadequacy. In turn this may make him more demanding or prompt him to feel he is 'a burden' and 'far better out of it all?' Along with the patients families therefore will need pastoral care and support with a ready recognition and understanding of their problems and a full and sympathetic opportunity to express their grievances and frustrations.

It will be important not only for the family but for all who are concerned in a caring ministry to be familiar with the various resources which are available in both hospital and community, and it is to a description of these that the next two chapters are devoted.

Chapter 3

The Hospital Team

A large hospital can be an organism of bewildering complexity, with many differing skills and functions dove-tailing to fulfil its grand purpose. It is most important therefore to know what helps to make the hospital 'tick', and the various grades of staff who help run it. Pastoral ministry among the hospital staff will only be effective as the priest is able to co-ordinate his own services with those of others in the hospital team. He will attempt to be in touch not only with 'key' members of staff but also with all whom he may meet in the course of his visiting.

There are two main groups of hospitals—teaching and non-teaching. A teaching hospital provides tuition and training for medical students. The students receive their pre-clinical training at a university medical school, and their clinical training in the hospital, where members of the medical staff give them practical instruction in the diagnosis and treatment of diseases with patients in the wards and other departments. The teaching hospital will also have large training schools for nurses. The non-teaching hospitals comprise by far the larger group.

It is practically impossible to define hospitals in anything like specific terms but the average general hospital will deal with most kinds of disease encountered in the population, and provide facilities for general medicine, general surgery, orthopaedic surgery, ENT surgery, dermatology (skin disease), obstetrics (childbirth), gynaecology (disease of female reproductive organs), paediatrics (children's diseases), geriatrics (diseases of old age).

At the very centre of the hospital's main task will be the medical staff.

Medical staff
The medical staff of a hospital consists of a number of consultants, senior registrars, registrars, house physicians and surgeons. The *consultants* are in charge of all the medical work of the hospital, and all patients referred to hospital by a general practitioner for in-patient or out-patient treatment become the responsibility of the consultant. He it is who has to make decisions about their diagnosis, treatment, referral and discharge. He is helped by his junior doctors and by a variety of nursing and paramedical staff. In practice the *senior registrars* and *registrars* have some autonomy although they are responsible to their consultant. They in turn supervise the work of the *house officers* or *housemen* as they are commonly called.

The medical staff work together in small individual units called 'firms'. A 'firm' usually consists of a consultant, a senior registrar, a registrar, two or more housemen, and a number of medical students. Every consultant therefore has his personal team working under him, who are responsible for looking after all the patients admitted under the consultant and occupying an agreed number of beds in the various wards of the hospital.

When the patient is admitted to the ward he is examined by the houseman who writes up a medical report in the patient's case-history. Later on the registrar will examine the patient and detail the houseman to see to various procedures, if they are deemed necessary, such as X-rays, blood-tests etc. Finally the consultant will see the patient during what is referred to as 'the ward round', when he is accompanied by his registrar and housemen, the ward sister and one or two senior nurses. In the teaching hospital medical students will also form part of the retinue. Should the firm be a surgical one discussion will take place about operating sessions and lists, and which of the operations the consultant will perform himself and which will be entrusted to his registrar. The consultant *anaesthetist* will be responsible for the administration of the anaesthetics at the operation and he and his colleagues will visit all the patients listed for surgery and study their case-notes, and if necessary make their own examination. The anaesthetist will explain to the patient what is going to happen on the day of the operation and how the anaesthetic will be administered, thereby reducing any feeling of tension and anxiety.

The medical staff do not treat patients in isolation and receive various forms of assistance from a number of different members of other hospital staff which can be termed paramedical. Paramedical staff are not involved in the central tasks of diagnosis and treatment but rather help the doctors perform these functions.

Nursing staff

Nursing ranks are indicated by various types and shades of uniform and these differ from hospital to hospital. The present nursing management structure is known as 'Salmon' after the name of the chairman of the committee set up in 1963 by the government. The committee's report noted that the well-known title of 'matron' applied equally to nursing heads of hospitals as small as 10 beds and as large as 1,000 beds, and that a distinction between their different duties and rights was not at all clear or well-defined. Again as men were increasingly becoming nurses the old titles of 'matron' and 'sister' were becoming anachronisms. It was also noted that nurses' roles as administrators were rather vague and open to confusion. The committee recommended that in future most senior nurses deciding policy be called 'top managers', those programming policy 'middle managers', and those controlling the execution of policy 'first-line managers'. The terms 'sections', 'units', 'areas', and 'divisions' were also introduced and senior nursing posts were named accordingly.

At the top of the nursing structure is the *chief nursing officer* (CNO) responsible for all nursing services and education in the group and not identified with any one individual hospital within it. The *principal nursing officer* (PNO) is responsible to the CNO for the management of a division—i.e. a large part of the nursing service or all the nurse training within a group. The *senior nursing officer* (SNO) is responsible to the PNO for the management of services within an area, which might be the whole of a separate medium-sized hospital or a number of small hospitals. The *nursing officer* (NO) is in charge of a unit, that is three to six medical or surgical wards, or for example, a small suite of operating theatres, a specialised unit or an accident and emergency centre. The nursing officer is in close touch with patients and is available for less experienced staff to turn to for advice in the absence of the ward sister or charge nurse. The *charge nurse* (male) or *ward sister* (female) controls an individual section, which can be a ward or an operating theatre.

There are various grades of nursing staff. The student nurse is undergoing a three year training course to become a State Registered Nurse (SRN). In the psychiatric hospital she becomes a Registered Mental Nurse (RMN). The pupil nurse is being trained for two years to become a State-Enrolled Nurse (SEN). In some hospitals there are nursing auxiliaries, and/or nursing assistants (part-time) who are untrained staff but have attended induction courses.

The work of the different types of paramedical staff is extremely varied, but as a whole it represents an identifiable and essential component in the whole programme of clinical care, without which medicine and nursing would be of limited effectiveness.

Social workers

In the treatment and management of all illness the reaction of the patient to the various social factors which he faces—his family, his work—are often quite crucial. In those in which the illness is largely produced by the psychological reaction of the patient successful diagnosis and treatment are dependent upon the ability to understand, change or influence for the better, the patient's reaction and adjustment to these social aspects. The unravelling of many of the more complicated social features in disease is undertaken at the request of the consultant by a trained *social worker*. In the reorganisation of 1974, the control of hospital social workers was transferred from the health services to local authority social services departments. Their work in all its aspects forms part of a team approach and assists and complements that of the consultant and his medical team.

There are four main areas of work for hospital social workers.

The largest and most important aspect of hospital social work is *medical casework* which is concerned with the adjustment of the patient and his family to the patient's disease. It mainly involves working with the patient in hospital (including in-patient and out-patient work) but may also necessitate the hospital social worker visiting the patient's home. All types of cases are covered, work with children including non-accidental injury cases; much work is also undertaken with the elderly, many of whom live alone and are consequently very vulnerable.

Another group which is especially important to the hospital social worker is the longstanding or chronic patient especially if he has a disability. After the acute treatment of any such patient has been carried out, the next stage of successful rehabilitation back into the patient's own home and normal life (back to employment) may depend on solving as many social problems as medical ones. For instance mobility is of paramount importance for anyone who is going to return successfully to work. The hospital social worker is expected to know how these can be best dealt with and has the responsibility to arrange all the various solutions—special transport, industrial training, special housing etc.

Terminal cases are included, especially those patients who are suffering from carcinoma. Illness in the parent of a one-parent family often produces many extra difficulties which the hospital social worker will try to solve. Another important group of cases are accident patients and especially those suffering from chronic disabling diseases including rheumatoid arthritis. Many social problems occur in mental illness and the role of the hospital social worker in such cases is often a crucial one.

Environmental help will often be needed and the social worker will arrange how the patient's home can be improved to help him cope with his illness. This may involve the complete rehousing of the patient or the adaptation of the home either structurally or by the introduction of certain aids. It is most important that the inevitable problems are considered early enough to enable a satisfactory solution to be worked out by the time the patient is ready for discharge. The hospital social worker will anticipate difficulties by arranging with the corresponding local authority social services department to order the necessary structural work or aid required as soon as possible after the need becomes firmly established.

Arrangements will be made for *immediate assistance to the patient or his relatives*. A further function of hospital social workers could be classified as arranging features which *facilitate medical care*. It includes a wide range of functions many of which might be described as routine or superficial service for patients and their relatives which do not involve social case-work. These include financial help, convalescent arrangements, provision of escorts and accommodation for relatives.

Another important function of hospital social workers is the necessary *liaison work* between the team in the hospital treating the patient; doctor, nurse, physiotherapist, occupational therapist; and the various other statutory and voluntary agencies working in the community. Most of this liaison is with the social services department of the corresponding local authority, for this department acts as a necessary link between the hospital services and the community social services. Many of the facilities required by patients either in the form of services, aids, and adaptations, telephones, are initiated by the hospital social worker contacting the social services department who then provides the service required.

Administrative staff

Administrators in the National Health Service manage institutional and support services, provide administrative services and act as general co-ordinators. The health services are now so comprehensive that administration has a vital role to fill, for it has to see to the efficient co-ordination of the many occupational skills represented in health care— doctors, nurses, dentists and opticians, and of the therapeutic services, scientific and technical services. The management service with its computer operators, analysers and programmers, and with its specialised techniques of ward study, organisation and methods, programme budgeting and similar aids to offer help to effective management, all play a significant part in administration.

There are also officers in charge of other essential services. The *catering officer* is responsible for the ordering of supplies for his department, budgeting and cost control. He is in charge of the kitchen, preparation of meals and menus and their distribution and service. The *dietician* recognises the importance of food and patients' feeding habits and customs. She advises the catering officer on planning menus which provide suitable food for patients at different stages of their illness. She also carries out important work in the diabetic and metabolic clinics or units. The *domestic services* are responsible not only for cleaning the various areas of the hospital, but also for the smooth running of a range of housekeeping activities, the correct treatment and maintenance of floors, furnishing and fittings. The staff look after the services in the wards, reception areas and clinics. The *occupational therapist* works with doctors, nurses, and other members of the team, helping patients to recover mobility and skills, and to return to active life in the community. Patients are referred to the occupational therapist by a doctor, and most work is done in general and psychiatric hospitals and rehabilitation centres. The department often includes a workshop and facilities for industrial or clerical work training and domestic rehabilitation. The *radiographer* works under the direction of a radiologist. Her main function is to position patients properly so that there is a correct definition of bones and organs, and to take the X-ray pictures not only in her unit but also in operating theatres and wards. Therapeutic radiography provides treatment by X-rays and by radiation from other sources such as radium and radioactive isotopes. Apart from the mobile mass X-ray units, radiography is a hospital based service. The *physiotherapist* treats the injured or diseased by physical means, exercises, including exercises in water (hydrotherapy), manipulative techniques, and thermal and electrical procedures. She will also be concerned with assessment of the patient's physical disability and will help the disabled to return to an active, independent life or enable them to cope with their disability. Treatment follows referral from a doctor, and, as with many other state registered professions, physiotherapists undertake to treat only those who have been so referred. *Remedial gymnasts* are concerned with the treatment and rehabilitation of patients through active exercises. Special apparatus, games and exercises may be used, following medical diagnosis and referral, for a range of conditions including functional training in perparation for work and special work with mentally ill and handicapped patients.

Engineers, electricians, ward receptionists, porters, telephonists, secretaries and *typists* and many other members of staff all play a vital part in the life of a modern hospital.

Chaplains

Every hospital should have a *chaplain* from each of the three main religious denominations, Anglican, Roman Catholic and Free Church, 'to provide for the spiritual needs of both patients and staff'. The majority of hospital chaplains are part-time (some 6,000), which means they are based in their own churches in the community and so can give only a limited amount of time to chaplaincy duties within the hospital. There are approximately 170 whole-time chaplains, the majority of whom are Anglican by religious denomination. Both whole-time and part-time chaplains are officially appointed members of the hospital staff, although the former have a greater opportunity to become integrated within the hospital community.

The role and function of the hospital chaplain have become more and more comprehensive and community oriented in recent years, for outpatient and day hospital and hostel facilities are greatly expanding and many patients, living at home, will continue their treatment on a basis of daily attendance at the hospital. His opportunities are widening and his relationships with other staff members becoming firmly established. Fortunately there is today a greater understanding of his ministry both within the hospital and outside in the community. Ideally the chaplaincy service should function as a co-ordinated and ecumenical team and the chaplains themselves recognised as essential members of the whole multi-disciplinary approach of health care. The very fact of the hospital chaplain's 'neutrality', in so far as he is separate and distinct from the various hierarchies in which all other disciplines working within the hospital are involved, and has no subordinates nor superiors, gives him a greater freedom to be concerned with the individual patient as a whole person and with the broader issues of the corporate health of both hospital and community. On the other hand his very independence makes it all the more imperative that he ministers in close co-operation with other disciplines and establishes good working relationships with all his colleagues. It is vital that he works in a satisfactory relationship with the medical staff, for his ministry is complementary to that of the doctor as part of the total care of the patient. A positive co-operation with social workers is essential for each will have much to contribute to the others' approach and case-work. The chaplain has also to win the full support and confidence of the nursing administration, ward-sisters and ward staff. Such co-operative relationships are mutual for all disciplines working harmoniously together contribute to and receive from each other the essential components for total health care.

The centre of the chaplain's work will be his ministry to patients, providing care and support by his sacramental and pastoral approach and sustaining and strengthening them in periods of crises. He attempts to provide 'meaning' for the patient in his present predicament, and by counsel, prayer and/or sacrament provides support and comfort. He is always 'on call' and respecting the privacy of the patient makes known his availability and accessibility. As chaplain he does not proselytize but is present to visit and counsel those who on their own initiative or his appear to need or to be ready to receive his ministry, for his primary concern is that of extending a relationship. Daily he has to wrestle with the basic issues of life and death, contradictions, meaning-lessness, guilt and estrangement, loneliness, anxiety, fear, despair and futility. Such feelings comprise the essential components of religious concern, and the questions they raise cannot be fully grasped apart from a religious understanding.

As well as ministering to patients the chaplain also endeavours to exercise an adequate pastoral care of families, staff, medical personnel and students, initiating and cultivating pastoral and professional relationships on a consistent, continuing and systematic basis of visitation and ministry. It is important, too, that while other disciplines are concerned about ethical issues and *may* raise the kinds of ethical questions that are important to quality of treatment and recognition of human need, the chaplain *must* raise those issues, and it is that compulsion that makes the chaplains more conscious and sensitive to these ethical issues and to bring them to the fore in deliberation of treatment teams.

Voluntary organisations
The tradition of voluntary effort in the hospital service is a long and successful one. Many hospitals now employ a Voluntary Services organiser to co-ordinate the work of a very large number of volunteers. *The National Association of Leagues of Hospital Friends* play a leading voluntary role in the hospital service. Three out of every four National Health Service beds are served by affiliated Leagues of Friends. These Leagues have a total of nearly half a million members, of whom 80,000 work actively in one way or another for their hospitals. They help in-patients and out-patients, and among their aims are the encouraging and fostering the interests of the public generally in the various activities and work of the hospital. They provide funds for both staff and patients, and help to recruit voluntary workers for local hospitals. Leagues of Friends also help to provide amenities and equipment which are not normally met by the National Health Service—e.g. the provision of major pieces of sophisticated and expensive medical equipment, and major amenity projects.

The Women's Royal Voluntary Service (WRVS) undertakes non-medical welfare work in some 1,225 hospitals throughout the country. The most widespread service is the provision of shops and trolley shops, and canteens for in-patients and their visitors and for out-patients. WRVS escorts help in out-patient departments of a number of hospitals. Patients are welcomed, escorted to different departments and in general given guidance and reassurance. The WRVS work in psychiatric hospitals and hospitals for the mentally handicapped is similar to that done in general hospitals, with trolley shops, canteens and diversional therapy.

The British Red Cross Society is an independent, voluntary organisation, whose principal task is to alleviate suffering among the sick, the handicapped and the frail elderly. It carries out its work through it voluntary unpaid members, who provide the following services in hospitals throughout the country—help with nursing duties, help with reception duties, creches for out-patients' or visitors' children, out-patients' and visitors' canteens, trolley or other shops, telephone trolley services, book library, picture library, beauty care, and help with other general duties.

Other well-known voluntary organisations such as Rotary, Toc H, Jewish Ladies Visitation Committees, Legion of Mary, Society of St. Vincent de Paul, are all actively involved in splendid work at local hospitals and play a vital role in the care and welfare of both patients and their families.

Finally, it must be emphasized that the most important member of the hospital team is the patient himself. Without him the hospital would be unable to fulfil its task of healing the sick. He should therefore be respected as a person who happens to be a patient and not as a patient who happens to be a person. So easily, amid the complexity of hospital life, can he be seen as a 'case,' a 'statistic' or a 'percentage', and be treated with paternalism and condescension. His dignity as a person must never be lost amid the intricacies of in-numerable administrative routines and medical procedures, no matter how efficient or skilled they may appear to be.

Chapter 4

The Community Team

Approximately ninety per cent of all illness is cared for at home. Hospital and community services are complementary components of our comprehensive health care. The hospital is a part of the community, and the community should play a vital role in the life and support of the hospital. Unfortunately the two words are frequently used in antithesis rather than seen as parts of a continuous process of health care. The average stay in hospital is becoming shorter and shorter, which means that comparatively few patients in acute district general hospitals need prolonged basic care. An increasing number of patients are being discharged soon after surgery to the continuing care of the community team. The number of patients attending out-patient clinics has increased considerably.

The primary health care team in the home situation is of course much smaller than in the hospital and its most important component is the family. In hospital there is very little opportunity for the team to get to know the whole person and care may be somewhat fragmented. The community team have the advantage of seeing the sick patient as a whole person in the context of his family and in his normal environment. Some of the social and emotional problems so easily concealed in the clinical setting of the hospital become far more apparent and obvious in the home and community. Prolonged contact and visiting allow a deeper and often a more honest relationship than is usually possible in hospital. Community care of the sick and elderly is a team activity.

There is the *general practitioner* who is responsible for most of the medical care provided within the National Health Service. On present averages about one in ten of the population can be expected to be admitted to hospital within a single year, but about seventy five per cent will consult their general practitioner and that about four to five times a year. There are about 24,500 G.P.s who each provide the full range of services to, on average, 2,307 patients. The people most frequently seen by a G.P. are the young, the old, and people living alone, and certain occupational groups such as miners attend more frequently than average. It is estimated that the G.P. is the first point of contact for about ninety per cent of people seeking treatment for ill-health, and about one in three of his patients will receive some form of hospital treatment each year. An increasing number of doctors now work from health centres, which provide an ideal base for the organisation of community care. The Department of Health and Social Security has exercised much flexibility in the size of health centres and in the number of general practioners working there as well as in the scope of community health services provided. The usual number of doctors working in a centre is between four to six with a full integration of health visitors, community nurses and school nurses. A unit such as this would undertake most of the community health services of the area.

The *community nursing team* comprises health visitors, community nurses and midwives who form a multi-disciplinary team working together in partnership with the general practitioner.

Health visitors are registered nurses with midwifery experience and a post registered qualification, and the essential part of their work is health education and preventive health care. They are under statutory obligation to visit every baby born in their area or registered with the general practice to which they are attached, and will continue to watch over the child's health and development until he or she reaches school age. Health visitors will also be concerned about the health of the members of the family unit as a whole, visiting them regularly and assessing their health needs. They will offer their advice and counsel where necessary and mobilise the resources of other services whenever circumstances arise. Part of their work will also include visiting mothers' clubs or clubs for the elderly, ante-natal classes and schools. Indeed they cope with certain aspects of physical, social and emotional problems of the community from birth to death. As a result of changes in legislation it became possible, from 1st January 1973, for men officially to enter the field of health visiting.

Their work as members of the community team may be summed up under five main aspects.

The prevention of mental, physical and emotional ill health and its consequences.

Early detection of ill health and the surveillance of high risk groups.

Recognition and identification of need and mobilisation of appropriate resources where necessary.

Provision of care; this will include support during periods of stress, and advice and guidance in cases of illness as well as in the care and management of children. (The health visitor is not, however, usually engaged in technical nursing procedures.)

Health teaching.

Community nurses (formerly known as 'district nurses'), like the ward sisters in hospital, are responsible for deciding the nursing care each patient at home needs and seeing that it is carried out. The patient in his own home with his family is a very different proposition from the patient in bed in a hospital ward, and the community nurse enters each home by the courtesy and permission of the respective patient or relative. They have no right of entry. Patients are normally referred to the community nurse by general practitioners, hospital liaison officers, social workers, health visitors or relatives. The first visit to the home is always paid by the state registered nurse who is the team leader, and assesses the situation. Later she may return and nurse the patient herself or she may delegate.

The present pattern is to attach community nurses and health visitors to a particular practice of general practitioners, and together they comprise the 'primary care team'. They normally work from health centres and doctors' surgeries. Ambulant patients are asked to visit the surgery for routine injections and dressings etc. Patients nursed at home have a twenty four hours a day and seven days a week service, exactly as if they were being nursed in hospital.

Night nursing services from 10.00 p.m. to 8.00 a.m. are available, as well as a night sitter service for patients who are very ill. A laundry service is provided for incontinent patients, and medical loans provide valuable contributions to the care of patients such as back rests, bed pans, urinals, bed cradles, wheelchairs for short term cases. Disposable equipment is used whenever possible as this lessens the risk of cross infection.

The domiciliary midwife, like the health visitor and the community nurse, is required by law to have undertaken specialist training and is qualified in the care of mothers before, during, and immediately after the birth of their babies, and in the care of the new born baby. The midwife is responsible for the care of mother and baby until the health visitor's responsibility begins, (usually when the baby is ten days old), although arrangements are normally flexible, varying according to each mother's individual needs. Midwives and health visitors may also share the responsibility for ante-natal teaching. The early discharge of patients after hospital confinement these days has resulted in many more puerperal visits being made by the midwife.

There are the comprehensive social services provided by

all major local authorities (county councils and metropolitan districts and London boroughs) under the Local Authority Social Services Act, 1970. This legislation follows the report of the Seebohm Committee published in 1968. Each authority has a Social Services Committee which controls services and in each authority there is a *director of social services* who is the chief officer in charge of the Department of Social Services. The following are the services provided by the social services department.

Care of the elderly (excluding medical care), including residential care, day-care services such as clubs, meals on wheels and social work support.

Care of the physically handicapped (excluding medical care)—the blind, deaf, spastic, epileptic, and paraplegic cases—including residential and day care.

Care of the homeless (temporary accommodation).

Child care protection, including child care supervision, acceptance or parental rights of children committed into the care of the local authority, control of children's homes, admission units, reception centres, social work support and certain adoption services.

Social work and family casework with the mentally disordered, including provision of social workers (formerly mental welfare officers). Also included are day centres, adult training centres, workshops and residential accommodation (hostels) for the mentally disordered.

Day care of children under five years of age, day nurseries and child minding.

Provision of home helps.

Care of unsupported mothers including residential care.

It is of vital importance that the closest links possible be maintained between all medical and social services. A number of the social services represent the main supporting services within the community for those persons recovering from illness or suffering some chronic disabling condition. Both health and social services are now generally organised over the same geographical areas, following the reorganisation of the health services and local government in 1974. It is hoped that local arrangements are made to assist day to day co-operation between the two important services. Links can be established between social workers and the local health centres and group practices, and good working relationships fostered with social workers and local hospital services particularly at geriatric and psychiatric hospitals. It is of prime importance that there be a strong liaison of social workers with health visitors for they will be dealing with a number of mutual problems albeit from different aspects.

Local churches also play an important role in community care. The sick at home will be visited regularly, the lonely befriended and the anxious family relieved of much strain and stress. Communicant members of the congregation will be brought the sacrament at home, and be continually upheld and enveloped into the life and worship of the community in eucharist and prayer-group. Members of local church organisations will help patients living alone over the first few difficult days after leaving hospital by airing beds, preparing meals, shopping, lighting fires and offering much general practical help. Whenever possible the chronically sick and disabled will be taken out for a drive or to church where they will once again feel part of the worshipping community.

Good-neighbour schemes will be organised by local churches making arrangements for those who live near the elderly, the lonely and the house-bound to call in regularly to help with simple domestic chores—lighting fires, cooking, shopping, light housework. Merely 'calling round for a chat' is also a much appreciated service to the friendless and lonely, particularly those who have recently been discharged home from hospital after an illness.

It is the duty of every social services authority to provide a *home help service* adequate for the needs of the area. The work of home-helps in the majority of instances is with the care of the elderly but other groups are also covered, including maternity cases and acute or chronic illness as well as the younger physically handicapped. Normally a charge is made for this service but there is a sliding scale according to income. For those who receive social security or old age pension as their only income the service is free. Obviously their duties will vary considerably but will include most of the normal tasks carried out by a housewife—preparing food and meals, cleaning, ironing, shopping, lighting fires, looking after children. Dependent upon the family circumstances home-help service can be provided full-time or part-time.

Ideally the home-help will form part of a co-ordinated social work team and work co-operatively with social workers in the area, for she will have much to offer to the fullest possible social support of the families concerned. She will have become aware of various social or emotional problems in the households she serves, and for this reason will seek to liaise with the general practitioner, community nurse and health visitor.

Meal services include the meals-on-wheels service which provides a hot, two course meal delivered to the home of an elderly and/or sick person usually as often as the need arises. Some of the less frail elderly will perhaps be able to attend *luncheon clubs* at a local club or church hall and there obtain a hot meal. The added advantage of such a setting will be the companionship of others as well as the regular exercise involved in walking to and from the local centre.

One of the most critical times for a number of old people is when they are discharged home from hospital after an illness, for when living on their own they become particularly susceptible to rapid deterioration. At such a time *home-care programmes* provide home-help and meals services plus home nursing services for the elderly recently discharged from hospital for at least four weeks following discharge. Consultants and hospital social workers select the cases to be helped and give at least one week's notice of discharge so that the home-help and other services can be waiting for the old person on discharge from hospital.

Day centres provided by Social Services Departments,

Area Health Authorities, and voluntary bodies, organise recreational and treatment services, e.g. chiropody, activation therapy, occupational therapy, health education and meals for elderly people during the day time. Regular transport is provided to collect the old person from home to take him to the day-centre in the morning and home again in the evening. Day centres are particularly helpful for old people living with relatives who go out to work, or for those who live alone.

Large well established *voluntary organisations* provide a wide range of welfare services both on a national and a local basis—The British Red Cross Society, Women's Royal Voluntary Service. For example, owner-drivers play an important part in taking out-patients to hospital for treatment through the hospital car service. This important service is organised in conjunction with the Ambulance Service jointly by the St John Ambulance Brigade, British Red Cross Society and WRVS, each being responsible in different countries.

The term 'voluntary organisation' covers those non-profit making associations which are not created by statute. The contribution of such organisations alongside the statutory provision of health and social services is considerable. They can often identify particular areas of need and specialise in educating public opinion on the deficiencies and potential improvements in statutory services.

Voluntary societies also include a number of specialised services, e.g. the NSPCC, National Children's Home, Family Welfare Association, as well as groups dealing with the elderly such as Age Concern, and those working in the field of the disabled, including the central Council for the Disabled and the British Council for the Rehabilitation of the Disabled. There are also self-help groups made up of people who suffer from a particular disability, and their families and relatives e.g. Alcoholics Anonymous, National Society for Mentally Handicapped Children, The Haemophilia Society, Multiple Sclerosis Society.

Community Health Councils were introduced into the

health services following the National Health Service Re-organisation Act, 1973. Their main function is to represent the local consumer's interests and to ensure that the development of local health services takes regard of local opinion, and to help the managing authorities by making them better informed on local priorities, needs and deficiencies. Each Community Health Council must admit the public to its meetings and ensure that the public is aware of the names of the chairman and members.

The matters with which the Community Health Councils are primarily concerned are as follows.

General effectiveness of the health service in the district.

Planning of health services.

Variation in local health services—closure of hospitals or hospital departments.

Collaboration between the health services and local authority social and education services.

Standards of services, i.e. number of hospital beds in the district, the average number of patients on family doctor's lists.

Patient facilities including hospital outpatients, open visiting of children, waiting times, amenities for hospital patients and arrangements for rehabilitation of patients.

Waiting periods for in-patients' and out-patients' treatment and for domiciliary services.

Quality of catering in hospitals and in other health service institutions.

Complaints—not individual patient complaints but the general type of complaint.

Advising individual members of the public how and where they should lodge a complaint and the facts that should be provided.

When the patient is sick at home it is the family members who shoulder most of the responsibility for his care and dependence. Indeed should the illness be chronic or prolonged the effect can lead to much stress and strain, and interpersonal relationships can be disrupted. The need for constant attendance can be very demanding. Members of local congregations can play a major role in alleviating the strain by organising night sitting services for example, and by their caring and supportive companionship and practical help.

It has already been emphasised that community care is a team activity and it is therefore vital that there be close liaison and full co-operation between health and social services in the total care of the patient. Such team work will also help to foster health education within the local community which should be the responsibility of every sect of society. To be effective, health education must influence the attitudes of individual people and therefore must permeate into the home, family life, school, work place and recreation.

The most effective method of furthering health education is by *personal* discussion between doctors and patients, health visitors, clergy, nurses and simple and practical demonstrations in the home. One of the key figures in *individual* health education is the general practitioner who has a knowledge of the family background and is someone in whom members of a household can confide. The parish priest or minister will work in full co-operation with the local doctor, for he will be someone who is aware of people's needs and relationships in home and family. The health visitor too, will have an understanding of the home and social environment and so have a personal contribution to make in the course of her day to day tasks.

Small groups who meet together regularly in schools, factories, or health clinics, gain much insight through study and discussion and the use of various visual aids (film-strips, films, colour slides). In *group* health education the individual gains much support and encouragement from other members. It is therefore important that the group be kept small so that maximum help is derived.

Mass media health education will help to teach the whole

community by means of radio, television, posters, etc. and it is important it be supported by both individual and group discussions. Finally, there are special health education campaigns tackling such problems as alcoholism, smoking, immunisation or accident prevention, mass X-ray, drug misuse. In tackling any problem there will always be two main objectives—*primary prevention* to reduce the likelihood of more people becoming involved in the particular problem, and *secondary prevention* to help those who are already involved from further deterioration of their condition.

For far too long has health education been seen as the sole charge of the professionals—the health educator, general practitioner, health visitor, community nurse, social worker. If it is to be successful it must have access to as many people as possible and will involve all sections of the community—parents, teachers, employers, youth leaders, church leaders, politicians—for it is everybody's business.

Chapter 5

The Various Needs (1)

It must be made clear at the outset that there can be no clear-cut classifications of various needs, for there are no standard patients, each being a distinct individual with his own unique personality. Each patient is a person with whom to be identified, a child of God to be loved, a member of the community to be respected. The priest should be cognisant of the fact that he is, first and foremost, an ambassador of Christ, in whose name he comes to minister in hospital or home. He will bring confidence and assurance in his bearing; he will bring poise and calm, for all about him may be disturbed and anxious. His personal prejudices and problems must be set aside so that he is free to concentrate on the patient as a person; his attitude must be receptive as well as responsive. All contacts with the staff in hospital and the family at home are to be cultivated, for the effectiveness of his pastoral care will depend upon good interpersonal relationships. The prayers of the priest before visiting the sick will help him to cultivate a sympathetic sensitivity to their various needs and resources; his notebook of intercessions will be his constant companion and prompt him to recognise their longings and be alert to their desires.

In the course of his sick visiting he must have insight into the needs of various types of patients such as the following.

The paediatric patient

One of the most important elements in the pastoral care of a sick child at home or in hospital is that of establishing a relationship in which the young patient recognises that he is seen as a person of worth, with his self-identity fully and openly acknowledged. He is not a little man or a little woman; neither is he a mini-adult. The priest and all who visit must understand the emotional states of sick children in general, and the special needs of each sick child in particular. They must be keenly sensitive to their own self-awareness, and of their own feelings when confronted by the pain and suffering of the young. Only then will they find themselves free to minister and be ministered to, to teach and be taught, to guide and be guided. The feelings of sick children are often quite spontaneous and unaffected by artificialities which makes it all the more exciting and challenging to be with them. Their honesty and frankness are refreshing traits and so much can be gleaned about the whole art of prayer by listening and noting how they express their personal feelings to God.

The priest will be aware of the several factors which influence a sick child's reaction to being admitted to hospital. The most common is the separation from its parents which will often be marked by bouts of crying and emotional upsets, as well as periods of pent-up fear and distress. The age of the child will also play a part, children of under school age being specially vulnerable to emotional stress. The length of his stay, the nature of his illness, previous experience of hospital care are other factors which have a bearing on his reactions to hospitalisation.

Much of a sick child's anxiety, fear, and stress can be alleviated by good inter-relationships between himself and other children and members of staff, and by effective communication through which he is helped to understand hospital procedures and gain confidence towards all who are ministering to him. Various medical procedures can often cause a child much fear and emotional distress, and if he does not understand what is involved he will often fantasize and imagine all sorts of fear-inducing and frightening experiences. Whenever possible parents should be included when staff explain medical or surgical treatments with the child. In this way, such communication will not only relieve the fear and apprehension of the child itself, but will also help the parents to become an additional source of comfort to him.

Those who minister must be keenly alert to the various meanings and interpretations a child gives to his illness. He may view it as a punishment for 'being naughty'. He may feel his parents are in some way responsible or at least should have been able to prevent it. Should he be in an open ward in hospital with a number of other sick children around him he will be taking careful scrutiny about what is happening to them. If some of the other children are very ill or having 'unpleasant things' done to them he will naturally be wondering whether the same will happen to him. In a hospital ward he will of course be separated from his familiar home environment, and it is important for the priest to have a sympathetic understanding of the necessary adjustments a young child has to make on admission to a strange and new setting. In his early days he may become somewhat confused and frightened by the unfamiliar surroundings. Under normal circumstances however it does not take him long to begin to take an interest in ward routine, to get used to white-coated figures attending him, and to make friends with other children on the ward. Fortunately these days parents are encouraged to stay with their children and many paediatric units have provision for mothers and fathers to stay on the ward should it be deemed necessary.

At the bedside, ministry to a sick child will include a sharing of his interests and involvement with his play-things. Often the way he plays his game or paints his pictures will give a helpful insight into his character and his emotional traits. Play is a most effective 'acting out' method of dealing with his anxieties and fears, and potentially traumatic experiences can often be anticipated. Generally conversation should be kept fairly brief for, dependent upon his age, his attention span is short. An effective relationship will depend for its meaningfulness not so much on what is said verbally but on non-verbal communication and relatedness. Children are extremely sensitive to the real self of those who minister to their needs, and are quick to tear away any veneer or facade. What makes visiting them such a joy and delight is their simple yet strong faith that all is going to be well, for they have a confidence and a trust to be envied and admired.

Emotionally disturbing fantasies about medical or surgical treatment can readily be conjured up in their minds, and strange and unfamiliar instruments, apparatus and objects can evoke much anxiety or panic unless some helpful explanation is given for their use. It should always be borne in mind that such fantasies are as real or more real, in some instances, to a small child as the world about him. Often the best way through to him will be an approach to the parents, who will need much supportive care and attention. They too have all sorts of problems and are naturally apprehensive about the physical well being of their offspring. For them it is a time of much stress. Mother may feel torn between her love for her sick child in hospital, her love for her other children at home, and her devotion to her husband. Each can have its separate pull, and place added strain on to an already anxiety-ridden mother.

Parents often experience feelings of guilt and ask themselves such questions as, 'Should I have sent for the doctor sooner?' 'Am I in any way responsible?' They feel they must have failed somewhere in their upbringing of the child. Often there may be hostility expressed, aggression shown towards nursing staff, or anger projected on God. 'Why does God allow things to happen to a young innocent child?' In his ministry the priest has first to understand the strain and stress of the parents of a very sick child, and help and encourage them to express their true feelings. The tensions of the situation amid the regulations of the clinical setting of a hospital may make some parents feel occasional visitors rather than constant and comforting companions to their children. They may experience fear that the illness of their child is far more serious than they have been told, or that the medical procedures will be painful or have dangerous side effects. Parental separation anxiety must also be taken into account and fully acknowledged, and every provision made for them to spend as much time as possible with their child. They should always be encouraged to let the child know when and why they are leaving his bedside rather than just disappear or creep away when he is asleep. Their sudden absence can be very frightening and upsetting and a sick child is better able to cope with a 'departure' than a 'disappearance'. Assurance should be given that they will be returning soon, so lessening the child's anxiety and enabling him to wait patiently for their next visit. The members of the family should be allowed to be the way they feel in any given situation, but it would be hoped that eventually they would be led to see in their present crisis an opportunity for growth and healing. One of the essentials of pastoral care will be for the priest simply to be there alongside both family and sick child and to let them know that he is concerned and understanding.

Members of staff and all involved in the care of sick children will also need support and encouragement, for they too will have periods of emotional strain and stress. A caring ministry and a readiness to be available at all times on the part of the priest will be much appreciated. He should encourage staff members to communicate their thoughts and their needs freely, and to share their feelings of helplessness and frustration. There is a school of theology to be found in every paediatric unit and the more readily emotional and spiritual problems and concerns can be shared and worked through together the more full, rich and rewarding our mutual ministry will be.

The surgical patient

Surgery is a unique human experience and arouses a plethora of feelings and emotions, including the fear of pain and death. 'Will the operation be successful?' 'What will they find?' 'Will they tell me the truth?' are questions which frequently occupy the mind. There may also be the dread of anaesthetics and the fear of possible unconsciousness, discomfort, and post-operative pain. Regression and dependency are common accompaniments of surgery which enforces an almost childlike and passive behaviour on the part of the patient. It is erroneous to assume that a sick person who is to undergo what is commonly termed 'a minor operation' will experience any less stress and anxiety than the patient being prepared for 'major surgery'.

The more opportunity the patient has to express and release pent-up feelings the better, and those who minister to his needs will listen actively and sensitively, without interjecting their own opinions of how the patient should think or act. They will create an atmosphere in which the sick person feels quite free to express himself without being belittled. Anxiety is both a common and a normal reaction to surgery and patients should be reassured of this. Such anxiety is, however, often concealed and suppressed, and while keeping up a outward facade of calm and composure the patient may be inwardly stressful and panic-stricken. Much can be done by a sympathetic and understanding approach to alleviate the distress associated with anxiety, even though the anxiety itself is not dissipated, and both verbal and non-verbal communication of the acceptance of the patient's feelings should be conveyed to him.

The feelings and emotional strains of a surgical patient will much depend on the specific part of the body involved, for his bodily image can be greatly affected by various surgical procedures. *Stoma surgery*, for example, can be a frightening and sometimes shattering experience for the patient concerned. He will often fear he will become a social outcast or never be able to live a normal life again, when a colostomy (a surgically established fistula between the colon and the surface of the abdomen), ileostomy (a surgically made fistula between the ileum and the anterior abdominal wall) or a ureterostomy (a permanent fistula through which the ureter discharges urine) is advised. It is often when the patient who has undergone such procedures prepares to return home that his problems become a reality; for he is away from the security of the ward with other fellow sufferers around him, and he fears that his family and others may not be able to cope with his difficulties away from the sheltered and skilled hospital community. At home he may wish to protect himself not only from his friends but also from his family and those near and dear to him. He will need therefore every possible support and understanding both in hospital and when he returns home, and must be allowed time to come to terms with himself and his fears and apprehensions. He should be given full scope to discuss the things which are in the forefront of his mind. He may possibly feel he is now 'different from others', 'socially unacceptable', 'dirty' and 'objectionable'. Pastoral care should aim at encouraging and helping the stoma patient to lead as normal, and as active a life as possible.

The *mastectomy* patient (surgical removal of the breast) will also need the same kind of support and encouragement for similar reasons, and be assured that breast cancer is not an invariable death sentence. Many of such sufferers are more likely to die of old age or of some other illness than from their cancer. Where surgery has necessitated an *amputation* of a limb, the whole symptomatology of grief and mourning will often come into play, for the loss of part of oneself, be it arm or leg or body function, may often produce similar reactions to that of a death, for one has been literally bereft. Patients undergoing *heart surgery* have anxieties all their own for 'a bad heart' has a subtle symbolic significance, and the danger is frequently amplified beyond reality. As in all surgery there is a relationship between the degree of pre-operative anxiety and post-operative recovery. Therefore, the more counselling, support and understanding given prior to surgery the better, with full opportunity given to the patient to articulate not only his fear about the operation, but also the anxieties concerning his past, his future, together with the meaning of life and death. It is most essential that he has someone, be it chaplain, parish priest or minister, doctor, sister, social worker or friend, with whom he can be free to share himself and express his real feelings. Much of his stress and anxiety can be alleviated if he knows there is someone at his side who really understands him, accepts him and will be with him when needed. It is important too for the family to be given help, encouragement and support.

The surgical patient in an *intensive care (therapy) unit* is in an environment which is strange, highly technical and clinical, and also devoid of the nursing staff with whom he was familiar when on the ward. The physical presence of the priest in the ITU will say far more than his spoken word and his visits should be brief. The patient is dependent physically and emotionally on those around him, and will need to be relieved of all the anxieties which build up within him and make him fantasize about what seems to be happening to him. His family too will be undergoing strain and stress because they seem to be so helpless and alone in the midst of strange surroundings, with their patient surrounded by machines, and undergoing constant treatment which they do not understand. Often they have to wait in visiting rooms for long periods wondering whether or not the truth is being withheld with regard to the patient's condition, or what else will await them when next they see the doctor or sister. They will need repeated and constant explanation and reassurance.

In his ministry to the surgical patient the priest will require a working knowledge of the patient's individuality and an assessment of his real person. He should be aware that his feelings will probably include embarrassment, guilt, bewilderment, anger, and fear of both known and unknown dangers. Very real and very frightening is the fear of losing control or of being unaware of his surroundings. It is true to say that most of these anxieties and fears are not transmitted by words so much as by non-verbal means, and those who help most are those who listen not only with their ears but also with their eyes. Not in every instance will the patient voluntarily acknowledge that he has problems or difficulties, and the priest and those who share his visiting must learn to recognise some of these hidden defences and deal with their manifestations discreetly and supportively.

It should be remembered that *pain* is never a physical problem alone. In caring for those who are suffering painful conditions, especially those in post-operative stages, the priest must be aware of the complex emotional states of those involved and his pastoral ministry should centre around the whole person, the hurt body in its totality. In long continued pain a patient becomes exhausted, and feels isolated, trapped and completely occupied by the pain. Anxiety is the most common reaction and often unreal fears of the worst cause a vicious circle of confusing moods. To combat such anxiety it is important for the priest to establish good communication with the patient as well as to establish a confident and caring relationship. Along with anxiety there may also be feelings of anger and resentment, and in long continued pain patients can readily succumb to feelings of persecution, for it is extremely difficult for them to distract themselves from it or to compensate in other ways. It was C.S. Lewis who wrote in his *Problem of Pain* that 'God whispers to us in our pleasures, speaks in our consciences, but shouts in our pain'. Those in pain can become introverted and bitter, and feel they are being forsaken and abandoned by those about them. It is not always easy to comfort and reassure them, and it will need a ministry of utmost trust, tact and patience before they can be gently led to an acceptance of their true condition. Many a patient will look for some adequate cause as to why he is in pain and may give way to depression and feelings of increasing guilt. In attempting to seek some reason he will become convinced that he must have done something in the past to deserve his suffering. Regression is another response when the patient attempts to revert to being the centre of all concern, and looks for attention, and makes demands for help.

Perhaps the emotion most common to surgical patients is fear, a fear of the unknown and of surgery itself. The possibility of death seems always to be lurking on the sidelines, and in itself becomes a further cause for fear. The pastoral care of the surgical patient offers therefore a special challenge to the priest and all who minister to his needs.

The cancer patient

Cancer probably arouses more fear than any other disease. For the majority of patients it appears to be synonymous with death and much emotional strain is placed upon both the patient and his family. Fortunately early diagnosis and modern treatment have changed this grim picture substantially. Today many patients with cancer can be cured. Others have their lives extended and made more comfortable by advances in therapy. New advances in therapy are changing the old attitudes toward the disease.

Probably there is no one best way of answering the question, 'Should the patient be told?' Much will depend upon the patient's personality and his ability to cope with crisis and stress. Determining beforehand how the patient is likely to respond is the problem. A matter of particular concern involves communication among all who minister to the cancer patient. Evasion and subterfuge are common and these attitudes lessen the patient's confidence in those around him. The priest should not avoid his questions and concerns, for the patient should always be allowed to express them without being interrupted or having the subject changed. He should also have a clear understanding of what others, particularly the doctor, have explained to the patient. Ideally such matters should be regularly discussed among all who are ministering to the patient. Sensitivity and judgement are required concerning what is told in order to promote his comfort and well-being. All who care must do all to further the patient's trust in them and to help him to understand and deal with his illness, in accordance with the patient's values and his emotional and spiritual resources.

The diagnosis will mean different things to different people. Some will be completely overcome by the news and appear dazed and shocked; feelings of hopelessness, apathy and hostility will effect others, together with feelings of guilt and self-blame. A number of patients will speak quite openly about their condition, while others will dread the very word 'cancer' and suppress any painful or destructive thoughts from entering their minds. Defence mechanisms are frequently used to defend patients against their inner fear and anxiety, such as denial, dissociation, identification, regression and sublimation. By denying their real condition they protect themselves from the unpleasant reality by refusing to recognise it or face up to it. There is also a tendency for patients to identify with other people they have known who 'have had the same sort of thing'.

In the book *A Private Battle* (New English Library, 1979), which Cornelius Ryan worked on in total secrecy for over four years while writing his *A Bridge Too Far* and during which time he was told that he had cancer, he reveals openly his personal reactions to the diagnosis (pp. 20, 21). 'What comes to mind immediately is how fast cancer alienates one from the usual routines and behaviour. I suppose I'm less alive than I was yesterday and by tomorrow I'll be dying more than I am today. . . . I feel such a terrible sense of injustice. What did I do to deserve this?. . . . My mind swings from disbelief to fatalism. I am vacillating between a surging belief that all will be well and a maudlin conviction that nothing will ever be right again'.

In order to establish a meaningful relationship with the cancer patient the priest must needs be a good listener and have come to terms with his own feelings about cancer. He must be at ease with the fears, unexpressed as well as expressed, of the patient and be sufficiently skilled and tactful in enabling him to discuss these whenever the need arises. He must be able to feel with and yet be detached from the patient's emotions and anxieties if he is really to be sensitive to his needs and at the same time free to help. By conveying a caring attitude those who visit will enable the patient to communicate his fears and concerns. A non-directive approach of reflecting feeling, and restating of key words will reflect the visitor's sensitivity and integrity. He will try and see the illness from the patient's point of view and so gain an understanding of the patient and his concerns. Where he appears to be physically incapacitated or emotionally overwhelmed it may be necessary to speak slowly and distinctly, for a patient can become very frustrated if he feels he is being misunderstood or not given time to make what he feels to be a satisfactory response.

The continuity of care between the hospital chaplain and the parish priest and his people is of vital importance but unfortunately is not always fully recognised. Present day tendencies even for terminal patients are towards short in-patient care coupled with longer out-patient care, so as much liaison between hospital and home is essential. That there should be well defined and workable lines of communication between the local hospital and the church in the community cannot be over-emphasised. Frequent pastoral calls will give reassurance and a sense of security. It is most important for the priest, along with others, to help the patient maintain dignity and equanimity. Perhaps in no other disease is there such a threat to the concept of 'wholeness' as exists in cancer. The specific role of the priest and those who assist him will centre around the support of the patient in facing up to his illness and in creating an atmosphere at the bedside in which even painful truth can be discussed in an openness to reality. Apart from spiritual crises there may also be other crises peculiar to certain types of surgery and to particular treatments. Patients, for example, who have a colostomy or have undergone radical mastectomy may often experience much social and psychological embarrassment. These situations can have spiritual and emotional overtones of which the priest must be aware.

As a representative of truth and honesty the priest can give confidence and courage without glossing over the reality of death with superficial and banal reassurances. Through a ministry of sharing and caring, of presence, prayer and sacrament, he can assist the patient to live what period of time may remain to him with a sense of worth and dignity. He along with others can encourage the patient to gain a truer perspective on life and see that health is not the ultimate end of life. He can help the sufferer grope for values that transcend both health and survival, and so be ready to surrender himself up to a faith that can encompass even pain and suffering.

Prolonged pain can induce feelings of despair, rejection and loss of will to live. Wherever possible the cancer patient will be offered objectives for living, and given goals in life that may be meaningful and real to him. Where there is no sense of life, no aim, no purpose, the will to live soon becomes paralysed. Where the patient's will to live is encouraged and strengthened he becomes a fuller and richer person, a stronger and more complete individual; he is given a greater sense of self-respect, strength and hope. Where he has been helped to discover his own potential and to find and accept his own being, in his own time and his own way, his fear of death becomes diminished, although his physical condition may remain static or even deteriorate.

The attitude of the family is of prime importance, and pastoral care will include members of the family as well as the patient. There is a need for more resources and good-neighbour services to relieve families who are caring for patients in their homes. It is also necessary for the cancer patient to feel an important member of the local community right up to the end of his life. Attitudes and emotional states are contagious, especially where there is anxiety and regression.

Cancer has distinctive characteristics, and the very word strikes terror in the mind of almost every patient and conjures up a frightening, destructive spectre, unequalled in any other disease. It evokes an image not only of a fatal disease but one that devours and envelops from other directions, like the very derivation of the word itself—'a crab'. The closer and more important the person is to the cancer sufferer, the greater is the contagion or shaping of the other's state of mind. It is therefore of special importance for all who visit or care for the patient to avoid attitudes which imply or suggest fear, horror or helplessness. The most devastating of these negative attitudes is that of 'writing him off', or thinking of him as already dead. Such frightening fantasies and unhealthy reactions can unconsciously be communicated to the patient himself.

A great number of cancer patients are being cared for at home and receive help from the domiciliary services. It should be observed how the family are reacting. Do they understand the illness? Is there fear of contagion, which is very commonly held? Do they feel they always have to be doing something, which can often lead to an overindulgence of the patient? They can be assured of the importance of just being there, alongside the patient, of the necessity of communicating freely, and of showing compassion. They should do all they can to foster the will to live, for this adds a most important extra dimension to the traditional cancer therapies—surgery, radiotherapy, chemotherapy, and immunotherapy. Family members have a real need to give, to feel they are doing something of a practical nature to contribute to the comfort of their loved one, whether he be at home or in hospital. There can of course be no easy rigid rules for helping a cancer patient and his family, for each human being is different from any other. Each visit brings with it new challenges, new problems and new insights. Such a challenge however can provide a real opportunity to give and to grow. One theme will always remain constant and persistent—we must forget statistics when we care for the cancer patient and rather explore his inner and outer strengths and attempt to translate what is happening to him in terms of everyday living.

Chapter 6

The Various Needs (2)

The elderly sick

There are approximately 140,000 hospital beds (over one third of the sum total) occupied by patients over 65, and about the same number of old people resident in homes and hostels run by local authorities and voluntary organisations. By the end of the present century it is estimated there will be eighty per cent of beds occupied by the over 65. With increasing medical knowledge people today live much longer, and more of the elderly are finding their way into both general and psychiatric hospitals. Sometimes just a little patience and care would enable them to live a more active and agreeable life at home with their family.

It is important to study some of the physiological, sociological, and emotional factors involved in the aging-process. As old age approaches, abilities slow down. Losses, physical and otherwise, occur. Memory lapses and subsequent confusion become more prolonged. The impaired short-term memory of the elderly can make them uncertain of time and place. Old people become confused very easily when their environment is suddenly changed, for example, from home to hospital or from ward to ward. There appears to be a loss of recent memories, with a keen retention of past events and memories. There are also signs of decreased intellectual capacity, although human experience compensates for this. Interest in the world and in day-to-day living is reduced. Contributing to this may be many factors such as difficulty in hearing and seeing, which will prompt many an elderly person to become withdrawn and apparently uninterested. Cateracts are apt to form and often there is diminishing ability to focus on near objects. Advancing deafness is another symptom. Sometimes inability to hear causes a person to become irritated and angry, for anger is often born of frustration. Old age brings in its trail, too, a steady decline in motor function, and the elderly patient is inclined to move slowly and become prone to accidents. All these physiological factors tend to isolate the elderly from the community.

Social and emotional factors are of no less importance as the numbers of sick elderly people increase. Today there is a constant shift in family structure. Urban families are frequently uprooted and housed in skyscraper flats. Children grow up and move away, and those who do live near become more and more occupied with their work or with caring for their own families and have very little time to care adequately for their aged parents. Bereavement creates further isolation, for although there are many elderly who need to talk about their loss and work through their grieving they find few who are prepared to devote time to listen. Alongside loss of family there is also loss of work. Retirement can leave a life-long drive for work with no direction. Inactivity can be accompanied by a sense of guilt and a feeling of uselessness, of not being 'wanted' any longer. Consequently many of the elderly, particularly those who have no hobby or special interests, become depressed and unhappy. With a feeling of worthlessness they can suffer from identity-loss, and lose all desire to live.

With the growth of geriatric care as a speciality elderly patients can now be treated effectively in hospital either in a general medical ward which receives patients of many age groups, or a geriatric unit designed and run to meet the special needs of the elderly sick. There are also assessment wards where patients can undergo a range of physical and psychological investigations, diagnosis and treatment. Some patients may recover sufficiently to return home and do not necessarily have to become long-stay patients. The aim is to make full use of all resources available and to treat the elderly sick in the best possible environment by transferring them to the most suitable place or unit for their care. A large number will spend most of their time in the rehabilitation ward. Approximately ten per cent of all geriatric patients will be resident in long-stay wards, not being fit enough to return to their houses or even to the sheltered life of an old people's home. Here will be found the severely physically disabled who suffer from a variety of crippling diseases such as osteo-arthritis, rheumatoid arthritis, the after effects of a stroke, Parkinson's disease, multiple sclerosis and emphysema. Among the severely mentally and physically disabled patients will be those who have suffered a stroke or a form of dementia, whose features include disorientation, behaviour changes, intellectual loss and disturbance of normal personality. Unfortunately some long-stay wards and nursing-homes set aside for geriatric patients are unstimulating and monotonous. Ellen Newton in her book *This Bed my Centre* (Virago, 1980), which is her personal diary of six long years in a series of nursing homes for the elderly, pleads for the old to be treated as the living human beings they are. 'There's something so cold about mere passive acceptance', she writes. 'Probably the life-cycle of a flying beetle holds more interest and companionship than do the lives of the patients under this roof' (p. 22) '. . . In this less than half-world there are phases when time seems to freeze. Twenty-four hours don't mark one day. they stretch into an uneasy eternity' (p. 51).

Activity and interest are of paramount importance and social aspects of care are just as important as the physical and psychological. Where community care has been fully realised and encouraged, geriatric departments are able to extend their care beyond the hospital to the day-hospital which co-ordinates both home and hospital care. The day-hospital can serve to preserve, maintain and develop physical and social competence in the elderly sick.

In his pastoral care of the geriatric patient the priest together with his people must get to know the idiosyncrasies of the elderly and his approach should be as natural and normal as possible, with confidence and calm. Casual conversation can often prove difficult and frustrating for deaf patients cannot grasp quickly what is said to them. A deaf person should be spoken to slowly in a slightly raised voice with the words clearly enunciated. It is helpful to be in a good light so that if the patient is able to lip-read the mouth and lips of the speaker can be observed. Conversation can be elaborated by the use of simple actions and facial expressions.

Many patients are blind, and it is important to remember that they have no means of knowing who is approaching them until something is said. The priest and those who visit will help them, as far as is possible, to see that old age is far more than a negative state of being and that they can be creative in spite of failing physical powers. Often there will be much repetition in their conversation as well as a constant reminiscing about the past, yet they must be prepared to listen and so demonstrate God's love and interest. Many of the elderly sick have a simple yet sincere and strong faith with a deep sense of humility and serenity, and great patience will need to be exercised for they must not be hurried or given any sense of abandonment. The keynote of pastoral care will be reassurance and the instilling of confidence and encouragement. The more positive and practical the visit can be the better, and no matter how confused the patient may be his dignity as a person must always be strictly safeguarded.

There may often be opportunities for prayer or reading of familiar scriptural passages whose words are still treasured by the elderly and which bring much comfort. The Lord's Prayer and Psalm 23 will always be much appreciated. A number of the elderly will have lived sacramental lives in their respective home parishes and will treasure the sacrament of holy communion, for the reception of God's grace is not limited by physical capacity. Where there is regret, disappointment for sins and failings, the sacrament of penance will bring much peace and consolation. The priest should never be hesitant to express his own faith, neither must he be fearful of helping the elderly recognise the fact of death. Such a ministry will be a real testing of his own spiritual life and stability.

Lying in bed or sitting quietly in a chair the elderly patient can, if his physical and mental state allow, be helped to relax in his aches and pains, in his loneliness or isolation, and offer his whole being to God his Father in union with the pain and loneliness of his Son, Jesus Christ. He can offer his whole being on someone else's behalf, for those suffering alongside him and those who are ministering to his needs. In this way he will feel he is being used and given responsibility. Indeed he will often find that the day may not be long enough for all the things about which he may wish to think and pray. Old age affords a wonderful opportunity for silence, and the priest can often point to ways in which such periods of silence can best be utilised, and how in such moments the whole person may grow and mature and find God. Response and silence can produce peace, and what a reward peacefulness and tranquillity can be after perhaps long years of hard work and toil. As Jean Vanier writes in *Community and Growth* (Darton, Longman and Todd, 1979, p. 112) 'People who are old or sick and offer themselves to God can become the most precious members of a community—lightning conductors of grace. There is a mystery in the secret strength of those whose bodies are broken, who seem to do nothing all day, but who remain in the presence of God. Their immobility obliges them to keep their minds and hearts fixed on the essential, on the source of life itself. Their suffering and agony bears fruit; they give life'.

Approximately ninety per cent of elderly people live in the

community, so it is here that a great deal of pastoral care is needed. A large number of the elderly sick are looked after by their families often under stressful circumstances. A wide variety of social and other services are provided to help them function satisfactorily and also to help them maintain their independence. Such primary medical care is provided by the general practitioner, usually working in a group practice from a surgery or health centre. The team will normally consist of the health visitor, the community nurse, the midwife, auxiliary nursing staff, and in some circumstances a privately employed nurse and a social worker. They will work together, discuss individual cases and refer patients to the appropriate member of the team as necessary. Some health authorities run a night sitter service, which might provide holiday relief for a relative or support a family where the elderly person is particularly confused. Other services may include home help, meals on wheels, community occupation therapists, laundry service, telephone, chiropody, and library facilities.

The family of the geriatric patient will need much support and encouragement, for a great number of them will be sustaining heavy demands and often hospital admission will have followed years of devoted nursing care in the home. They will gain much strength from the fact that they are being supported not only by the prayers and intercessions of a caring community but also by the practical acts of service rendered. Some of the elderly sick become very irritating and demanding, and often react resentfully toward those who are nearest to them in relationship and are making much sacrifice on their behalf. This can be a very hard burden to bear for those who are doing most for them.

Members of staff, too, will be included in the pastoral care of the priest and his congregation. Although there are many joys and satisfactions in nursing the elderly sick there are also many strains and stresses. If members of the nursing and community care staff can feel free to discuss some of their feelings openly and freely they will at least be strengthened to face up to some of the more thankless aspects of their work.

Church congregations and parochial organisations can bring unique resources to help bring back the elderly into the mainstream of life and so strengthen a bond of corporate involvement. By their interest, attention and neighbourliness they can enable the geriatric patient to feel part of the life of the church, the body of Christ. By their frequent and regular visiting of the elderly sick they can break down much of the loneliness experienced by the elderly and add much to the zest of 'going on living'. It is estimated that over a million old people are living alone. Their needs are overwhelming and daunting. Some of the more mobile elderly can be taken for car-rides or transported to church services or to the local hospital when summoned for a medical 'check-up' or further medical investigations. Others might be invited into the homes of church members and made to feel one of the family. The housebound might be encouraged to make toys for a sale of work, knit squares for Oxfam, or crochet for a parish bazaar; for such a sense of belonging and of being used will all help to add significance to their lives.

It will be most important that the voluntary services provided by members of local churches see their function as *complementing* the work of the statutory services and not *competing* with them. Before undertaking practical schemes or projects it will prove helpful to contact the Social Services Department and the local Age Concern or Old People's Welfare Organisation so that resources are not wasted by duplication of effort, nor is the church seen to be working in isolation. The depth and intimacy of a caring congregation involved in the service of its elderly sick in hospital or at home can be a real fellowship of the Holy Spirit, for the christian gospel is all about love and relationships.

'It would be nice if we could go out on the crest of the wave and not via the geriatric ward', stated one elderly person. 'To go out *good*. Pray God let us do that. Go out good'.[1] To help

---

[1] *The View in Winter*, Ronald Blythe, Allen Lane, 1979. p. 314.

the geriatric patients 'go out good' is one of the prime functions of effective pastoral care.

The chronically ill

Ministering to the chronically sick patient provides many satisfactions and also poses some problems. Many will maintain a steady improvement while others again will remain static and even deteriorate. The chronically sick have significant problems in adapting to the restrictions imposed by their illness, and the very monotony of the routine, day by day, can prove discouraging. They are likely to be lonely for their illness appears not to be as dramatic as a critical condition, and they feel they are not receiving the constant and lasting attention they need. They usually have lots of time at their disposal throughout the day, and there is likely to be a tendency to brood unless they have some constructive activity to occupy their thoughts and fill up their time. There is, too, a likelihood of self-pity. Handicaps tend to frustrate, and frustration makes for resentment, and resentment is usually expressed in aggression. Aggression can readily irritate friends and visitors and discourage them from making regular visits. There is a danger among the chronically sick of them becoming 'institutionised' with a diminishing wish for recovery and a return home to face up to their responsibilities once again.

It is important to gain a genuine understanding of the condition and feelings of the patient. One of the prime tasks of pastoral care is to offer companionship to combat loneliness, and with regular visits to help keep the patient in contact with as much normal life and affairs as possible. The chronically sick should be shown how best their interests can be developed and cultivated so that they feel useful and needed. In this way they can be offered fresh rays of hope, yet be guarded from an over-optimism about their condition which may so easily lead later to acute bouts of depression. Both the families of patients and those who nurse them will need pastoral support for they are often involved in stressful situations which prove wearying and frustrating. They will need to feel they have a strong supportive and caring community behind them.

The critically ill
Considerable emphasis has been given lately to concepts concerning crisis and crisis intervention. Crisis can be defined in different ways. For some patients crisis means an experience during which their coping methods seem inadequate for the situation. Other patients will see crisis as a challenge—an opportunity or a turning point. The critically ill often have a fear of the unknown, as well as an inability to think clearly or rationally. Impatience can also be a common emotional reaction, with the patient becoming annoyed at the seeming calmness and casualness of doctors, nurses and others who do not appear to be treating his needs seriously enough. He may be in a comatose or semi-comatose condition with much of his conversation irrational, and his appearance have a stuporous look about it. One patient may be acutely depressed while another unduly optimistic. Some may wish to talk at length about their sickness and its symptoms while others may wish to remain silent and stunned.

The important thing to remember is that a patient is helped to deal with crisis by developing a feeling of competence. Too often his mood is one of helplessness. Some patients of course are helpless, either physically or psychologically or both, but by far the largest proportion of critically ill patients have considerable means of helping themselves but become so awed by the hospital and its strange environment that they feel unnecessarily unsure and helpless. Unfortunately many aspects of hospital care have a tendency to reinforce such feelings of inadequacy. It will be the task of the counsellor to find the patient's emotional level and begin wherever he is at that particular moment of time. He will avoid forcing his attention upon him, and should the patient want to talk he can be helped to express his fears verbally and freely. Under certain circumstances it might prove profitable to help him mentally face the worst possibilities that can happen as a result of his incapacity, for a new sense of strength and determination to meet any eventuality comes when a critically ill person has verbally met the worst. It is always better to express too little confidence than too much and the priest in exercising his pastoral care will be calm, composed and relaxed. Religious ministrations should be relevant to the situation and familiar to the patient thus helping him to develop a faith in himself, in others, and in God.

The orthopaedic patient

Feelings of extreme helplessness are common among patients whose mobility is seriously curtailed. It is important to distinguish between feelings of helplessness and actual helplessness. A patient with a broken leg or arm may be more distressed by feeling helpless than a patient in a body cast. It is essential to deal with the individual patient in relation to his response. The priest should help the patient to talk about his experience and enable him to express some of his feelings of powerlessness and if necessary to express his anger and resentment. Elderly orthopaedic patients will often despair of the future and the tasks of rehabilitation ahead of them; the young will be concerned about their education, their work and their family responsibilities. Anxiety over their disability is usually severe in young orthopaedic patients and threats to their body image and view of themselves as active, virile, and capable persons are very real. Anxiety over an illness becomes an additional emotional as well as a physical burden. Expressing feelings of anger, frustration or a sense of immobilisation in a disturbing life situation can effectively assist the orthopaedic patient with his physical ills and may even lessen the severity of his symptoms.

A loss of a limb can make a patient feel that he is less acceptable than others. It can lessen his self-esteem and affect his self-image. He can be expected to experience grief over his loss and, depending on his adjustment, he can normally work through the various stages of the grieving process. Not only can an amputation prove psychologically damaging but it may also create a number of difficult practical problems such as the possibility of lifelong invalidism, the loss of a job, and utter dependence on others. The loss of a limb may cause anxiety and grief even for the patient who has suffered long and severe pain. The entire response to amputation is highly individual and is affected by such factors as age, prognosis of the underlying condition, and the patient's emotional state and developmental level. Amputees need those around them who can help them cushion the emotional impact by the acceptance of their feelings and faith in their ability to cope with the problem. Patients should not be hurried through stages of grieving and need support to proceed at their own pace to integrate fully the experience. The amount of grief is usually proportional to the symbolic significance of the part amputated and the resultant degree of disability and deformity.

The pastoral care of those who are sick and in need will, it is to be hoped, be seen as an essential link in the chain of medical, surgical and total care of the patient. Amongst the various disciplines there should be mutual confidence, and a readiness to support, assist and learn from each other. There should also be a strong liaison with the community services and resources. To minister at the bedside of sick people both at home and in hospital, to watch with them, to learn from them, without of necessity knowing all the answers, is to symbolise our togetherness as a family. Such a companion-ship will surely prove a kind of redemptive presence that becomes in itself an aid to recovery.

Chapter 7

The Mentally Ill

It is important at the outset to differentiate between the two
conditions of mental illness and mental handicap for many
people confuse them and see them as one and the same
disorder. Mental illness can affect anyone, like any other
illness, but it can often be cured. Mental handicap is
something people are usually born with, and it cannot be
cured. Those who suffer from mental illness have special
problems with everyday living. The term 'mental illness'
covers very many states and in episodes of minor mental illness people become a liability to themselves, their families and
their neighbours. They seem unable to communicate rationally, unable to cope with certain situations, unable to work to
support their children, or they become irresponsible, or have
what is commonly known as 'a nervous breakdown'. Their
emotional states become unnaturally dulled or greatly
heightened and they become depressed, anxious or afraid for
no good reason. In its more severe forms it seems to affect
every respect of the patient's life and is often sufficiently incapacitating to necessitate admission to hospital. It can
make people withdraw into a world of their own; they cut
themselves off from reality, from their families, their jobs and
the society around them.

It is estimated that approximately ten per cent of the
population can expect to be admitted to a mental illness
hospital or unit at some time in their lives, and that one in
twelve males and one in eight females will enter hospital

because of mental illness at least once in their lives. Nearly half of all hospital beds in this country are occupied by people suffering from mental illness or mental handicap. There have been more and more people going into hospital because of mental illness over the past few years but this does not necessarily mean that psychiatric illness is on the increase. It means that more mental illness is now being recognised, more people are admitting they are ill and coming forward for early treatment. Of those people who are admitted to hospital nine out of ten leave within a year, half of them within one month. Many are treated as out-patients, living at home and coming to hospital for treatment at regular times each week. There are also a number of day hospitals which patients can attend each day for treatment and companionship returning to their families at night.

If the sick-visitor is to play an effective part in ministering to those who are mentally ill, whether they be at home or in hospital, it is imperative that he has a workaday understanding of some of the commoner mental disorders known as the neuroses, in which the patient's failure in adaptation is partial rather than complete, together with a knowledge of their treatments. Only the most severely disturbed neurotic patients, those who are unable to be cared for in the community, are likely to be accepted into a psychiatric hospital. Constitutional factors appear to be partly responsible in rendering the patient particularly vulnerable to stress. Often the illness is in some way related to traumatic experiences and to the parental attitude towards the patient in early childhood.

Fear and *anxiety states* are the most common mental disorders, presenting in exaggerated form all the physical symptoms which normally accompany any feeling of fear or apprehension in preparation for action. It is estimated that about five per cent of the population—over two and a half million people—suffer illnesses involving fear and anxiety. The majority are treated at home or as out-patients and the number in hospital at any one time is approximately 5,000.

The anxious patient complains of feeling worried and afraid, but does not know of what. Often he panics, anticipating the worst, and feels that some action is needed but does not know what it should be. He knows his fears are irrational and groundless but this is no help to him as he magnifies, scrutinises and mulls over the content of his anxiety. His concentration is poor and there is absentmindedness and insomnia and an exceptional degree of fatigue. The anxious patient is unable to relax, worries and frets over trivial things and tends to turn mole-hills into mountains. He may be intensely irritable and easily disturbed by noise; he may be afraid of losing a grip on things and to be 'going out of his mind'.

The causes of anxiety neurosis are many and varied. Some people by nature are more anxious and fearful than others. There is often an inherited predisposition towards insecurity, timidness, and emotional instability. Unhappy home conditions, domestic strife, poor social adjustments can also contribute to this condition.

The treatment of such states depends much upon tranquillisers, and also upon psychotherapy. Supportive psychotherapy seeks to relieve anxiety states by discovering causes in the patient's unconscious mental life, subscribing to the belief that behaviour is controlled by unconscious forces and emotion rather than by reason. Sedation may contribute to recovery by helping the patient remain calm and relaxed, while psychotherapy is an aid to better understanding by the patient of his problems.

Hysterical disorder or *conversion hysteria* is another neurotic state in which there is loss of function without organic damage, and is induced by stress. The patient is unconscious of the mechanism, and as the purpose served is clearly apparent to all others apart from the patient himself, the impression is often given that he is malingering. A psychological conflict is converted into physical symptoms involving one or more organs of the body making such disorders very diverse. Although the symptoms may be extremely incapacitating the patient appears somewhat complacent about his illness, because in fact the symptoms themselves represent the way in which he has solved an otherwise insoluble problem. Unlike the person suffering from anxiety neurosis, the patient with conversion phenomena is not obviously worried and indeed may deny worries; he is usually self-centred and likes to attract attention to himself. There are usually no deep emotions and feelings are inclined to be shallow.

As with the anxiety states treatment may consist of tranquillising drugs to calm the patient, followed by simple supportive therapy or prolonged psychotherapy to help the patient gain insight and a higher level of emotional maturity. Abreaction (a name given to a therapeutic process in which the patient relives a significant past experience which has contributed to the development of his illness, and benefits by such a discharge of pent-up feelings) is also used in the treatment of hysteria but is most successful immediately following some traumatic experience.

One of the most incapacitating mental disorders is *obsessive compulsive neurosis.* People who, prior to their illness, have often been known for their reliability, meticulous neatness, excessive concern for order, whose talk is precise, even pedantic and whose outlook is excessively moral and rigid, show these traits in exaggerated form should they become psychologically ill. They tend to have indecisive, vacillatory and hypochondriacal personalities, and lack imagination, creative ability and humour.

The process is an entirely unconscious one and occurs in two forms: obsessional thoughts and obsessional acts (compulsions). In the first process the patient finds it practically impossible to reach a decision over most straightforward matters because there is persistent doubting and the problem has to be considered from so many different aspects. He seems terrified to go out of doors, cross the road, travel by car or bus in case there may be a burglary or an accident. Fear of heights may be associated with an unconscious desire on the part of the patient to throw himself over. Other doubts may revolve around whether gas-taps have been shut off, or doors locked or whether an appointment has been forgotten. Such ruminations make life very difficult if not well nigh impossible.

Obsessional acts include repeated hand-washing and the expressed wish to be scrupulously clean. A housewife will have to make the beds many times over, wash up the same dishes repeatedly before being satisfied with the result. During periods of stress the patient's rituals may become complicated and so extensive that he is quite incapable of keeping them under control. Many sufferers from obsessive compulsions are intelligent people who fully realise the absurdity of their actions yet cannot fail but give way to them. For this reason to state the obvious to them only adds to a sensitive person's problems.

The treatment can be psychotherapy yet obsessional patients do not respond particularly well to this mode of treatment, as their pedantry and excessive concern with detail cause them to be enmeshed in the therapeutic process and brought to a halt. Some relief might be found by means of supportive therapy when pent-up feelings might be ventilated. Medication will take the form of tranquillising drugs to reduce anxiety, and whenever there is evidence of depression antidepressant drugs will be prescribed. In the presence of acute depression E.C.T. (electro-convulsive therapy) is found useful. In the treatment of chronic severe obsessional disorder accompanied by persistent tension and anxiety leucotomy (a surgical operation which divides the connections between the frontal lobes of the brain and the thalamus) is sometimes used.

In *depressive neurosis* there are states of sustained sadness or grief. In addition there are other bodily and emotional disturbances. A family bereavement may be a precipitating factor in some instances, although others will react to much more minor stresses. The accompaniments of depression are insomnia, loss of energy, loss of interest, weight loss. The depression itself can either be *reactive* (a fear and anxiety reaction such as loss of a job, examination failure, a broken engagement) or *endogeneous* (unrelating to external events). Depression is more commonly found in women than in men, and outbursts of crying are common. In the aetiology of depression age plays a part, and middle and old age are particularly vulnerable. Loneliness and the fear of death in old age and disillusionment in middle age are obvious examples. Rarely does it occur in adolescence but when it does it is inclined to be severe. To the depressive patient the world is dark, the future full of gloom and futility. He sees himself as an absolute failure—there may be forgiveness and hope for others, but certainly not for himself. Guilt and unworthiness are uppermost thoughts in his mind. All depressed patients who feel like this are likely to have suicidal tendencies, and threats should never be ignored. Deliberate taking of excessive numbers of tablets is common.

Fortunately depression is the most treatable of all the psychiatric disorders, and the majority of sufferers are treated as out-patients. Those who are acutely depressed, especially those with suicidal tendencies, have of course to be admitted to psychiatric units or hospitals. Good nursing along with sedation will help to alleviate some of the problems confronting the depressed patient, but the most effective treatment is physical and comprises of electro-convulsive therapy in severe states and also the use of anti-depressant drugs. Other helpful forms of treatment are supportive psychotherapy, occupational and industrial therapy and social rehabilitation.

Some of the more common psychotic disorders which in their severe forms affect every aspect of a person's life and are therefore often sufficiently incapacitating to necessitate admission to hospital include *manic depressive psychosis* in which elated periods alternate with phases of depression. In mania the patient is elated and feels on top of the world; everything is wonderful, and he is constantly active. He is inclined to speak rapidly yet without the usual logic, and punning and rhyming are very common. There is the tendency to spend money recklessly, to dress extravagantly, and to go from one project to another without completing anything. The patient has ideas of self-importance (delusions of grandeur) and over-optimistic views of life in general. These phases of mania or hypo-mania regularly alternate with phases of depression, but usually there is a period of normality in between phases.

The most common mental disorder which accounts for up to thirty per cent of all admissions to psychiatric hospitals is *schizophrenia*, a term used to describe a variety of disorders with certain characteristics in common but with considerable variations in other respects. The inner life of the schizophrenic patient is dominated by fantastic ideas; his emotional reactions are incongruous and he is so cut off from those around him that he appears to have withdrawn from the world. It is a most severe mental disorder which manifests itself in thought disorder, delusions, emotional disturbance, perceptual and behavioural disturbance. It is usually impossible to follow the conversation of the patient as it appears to be just a jumble of meaningless words and phrases, all totally unrelated. (This language is often referred to as 'word salad'.) At other times he seems to produce words of his own and these are called 'neologisms'. In addition to thought disorders there may also be thought blocking in which the patient's stream of thought is interrupted and a new line of thinking begins.

Delusions are defined as incorrect beliefs which are inappropriate to the person's socio-cultural background, and which are held in the face of logical argument. They appear suddenly and are held with strong conviction. They appear to be as inexplicable as they are incomprehensible. The patient may be convinced he is someone very important like a king or prime minister or a historical hero of the past. He may complain that the rays from the television are affecting his thoughts, his food is being poisoned, a plot is being devised to kill him or electricity is being passed through his body. He may find reference to himself in the daily papers, or programmes on radio or television. In all this he feels that his body or mind are under the influence of and being controlled by other people.

In severe schizophrenic states there is affective incongruity. The capacity for emotional response is greatly reduced and such emotional blunting means that there is neither elation nor depression and the outward appearance is one of complete indifference and apathy. It is therefore extremely difficult to identify with or empathise with a schizophrenic patient. Concerned as he is with his own private world he is totally unaware of things going on around him.

The most common perceptual disturbance is the *hallucination* which is defined as a false perception in the absence of any external stimulus. The patient hears voices which often sound unkind and say unpleasant things about him—that he is an evil person, lives a sinful life and is due for punishment. They may command him to do something and this often helps to explain his bizarre behaviour. As well as auditory there are also visual and tactile (touch) hallucinations. The patient may see monsters, evil spirits, or he is convinced he has insects crawling all over his body.

A schizophrenic patient's general behaviour will be very severely disturbed. States of ecstasy, wild excitement and impulsive behaviour are common, and drive is greatly diminished with a general loss of concentration. There is a strong resistance to suggestion which can express itself in stubborn behaviour or complete refusal to do anything. He may also act impulsively and race around in a state of extreme agitation or frenzy. He may adopt a statue-like stance for long periods of time without any apparent signs of fatigue.

Treatment of schizophrenia involves an eclectic approach for there appears to be no specific treatment for this condition. Psychological treatment would include individual psychotherapy wherever practical. More commonly used is group psychotherapy, yet here careful selection of patients is necessary. Social therapy would play an important role in the form of a therapeutic community. Chemical treatment includes the use of various drugs which not only calm the patient but also alter perception and modify his thinking. Electrical treatment is controversial but seems to be indicated when delusions and hallucinations are disturbing and giving rise to restlessness, overactivity or aggressiveness. Occupational therapy often proves invaluable, providing as it does a diversion from the patient's delusions and hallucinations as well as social contact with others. Activities such as art, music and drama classes give the patient an opportunity to express himself, and industrial therapy units provide meaningful tasks, emphasis being placed on making the situation as near to a normal work situation as possible. Such an environment prepares him for a return to the community when his condition improves sufficiently. Community care in out-patient clinics, half-way houses, and day hospitals all play a valuable part in helping in rehabilitation, and such care will involve hospital chaplains, social workers, local clergy and laity in collaboration with the hospital psychiatrists, general practitioners as part of a comprehensive community orientated health service.

There is only a thin veneer between the normal and the neurotic, and those who suffer from mental illness need to be sympathetically understood. It was Jung who once said that the most important thing about the neurotic is that he is so normal. Patients simply suffer from more exaggerated forms of emotional conflicts that are common to us all. In pastoral care they need to be met with a mixture of sympathy and challenge. What they need above all is a secure sense of belonging, a loving acceptance by other people. They experience much loneliness for they fear no one will take them seriously; they feel isolated and cut off from reality, and have a deep sense of guilt and shame. The basic enterprise in therapy is the quest for insight, and those who attempt to help must be able to listen, to learn to make sense out of the apparent non-sense of the mentally disturbed. To listen means to be interested in the other person; to be shocked or to condemn heightens the conflict of the patient. A human relationship in which he can be himself, without fear of rejection or exploitation, is like an oasis in a desert for the emotionally disturbed patient.

There are various ways in which the mentally ill can be helped, from an informal befriending to a more formal psychotherapeutic and counselling approach. Much will depend upon the experience and the training of those who are ministering to their needs. Ideally pastoral calls should result in one or all of the following accomplishments: a deeper knowledge of the patient, a clearer understanding of his problem, and progress towards helping to heal. The sincere observance of religious convictions and practices most certainly protects and safeguards mental health but it must be realised that religion is not a panacea any more than psychiatric treatment is an infallible means for curing a patient. Neither should religion be seen as a substitute for psychiatric treatment. In mental illness pious exhortations alone will prove but little help. At the same time it is entirely erroneous to consider religion as the hand-maid of psychiatry, for it has a mental health value all its own.

Those who are in the incipient stages of mental illness are often first observed by the priest, and he should therefore be responsible for doing something about them. Together with a trained group of lay helpers he can play a vital role in preventive care, and should be knowledgeable enough to know how to make an official referral if the situation demands. It is imperative that both priest and psychiatrist work in fruitful co-operation. The former should have sufficient appreciation of psychotherapy and the psychiatrist should show a sympathetic understanding of the patient's religious and moral needs.

Feelings of guilt are often prominent, and it is important to distinguish between guilt as rational judgement and guilt feelings. A normal person experiences feelings of compunction, remorse and shame, and these are usually in direct proportion to the sin committed and the objective extent of their guilt. In the neurotic person feelings of guilt do not always run parallel with intellectual insight, and are often out of all proportion to real guilt. Even after making an informal or formal confession the neurotic patient will be inclined to emphasise his guilt and feel more and more insecure and sinful. Both real guilt and pathological guilt will be worked through in cooperation with priest and psychiatrist.

One of the deepest roots of all neurosis, if not the ultimate cause, is a lack of being loved for what one essentially is, as well as lack of a loving acceptance of one's shortcomings and weaknesses. Neurosis is man's defence against the destruction of his true self. He thus becomes alienated from himself, estranged 'in the street' as Sartre has said. It is important that boundaries do not become confused between the roles of the priest and the psychiatrist, but it must be acknowledged that there will be many instances when lines of demarcation will be blurred and the two areas of pastoral care and psychiatry impinge the one on the other. No problem however need arise where there is a good working relationship between the various disciplines. Fortunately these days there is much mutual co-operation, understanding and respect between psychiatrist and priest. A number of clergy are now trained in the whole field of counselling, psychotherapy and group-work, and are generally regarded by the more progressive psychiatric hospitals and community resources as significant members of the treatment team. It is not necessary for all who visit the mentally ill to have a full and thorough knowledge of psychiatry, but it is essential for them to have a workaday understanding and to know the limits of each discipline. A little knowledge, if handled aright, is far better than none at all, and if sensibily used will not invite meddling. It is no great matter to obtain knowledge; the real test lies in knowing how to use it and in realising it is but a little knowledge.

Nothing helps to reintegrate a disturbed human person-ality more than acceptance. If the mentally ill are made to feel they are being accepted, just as they are, then this may have vitally beneficial importance for them. Those who visit them, either in home or in hospital, should learn not to be overwhelmed by their symptoms and mannerisms, no matter how strange and bizarre they may appear to be. Delusions and obsessions may seem totally irrational yet they are very real to those who suffer from them. In no way are they to be denied or above all ridiculed, but rather accepted as disguised expressions of deep-seated feelings and fears. Patience and an attempt at understanding will bear many dividends, for the need to build up trust and relationship is great. Those who attempt to help must not be over sympathetic nor wrongly submissive, neither should they see themselves as superior or outside the real needs of patients. There can be no 'we' and 'they' in ministering to the mentally ill.

In emotional illness the spiritual life of the patient is bound to suffer and often its immaturity or distorted features must be allowed to 'fall into the ground and die', before it can be nurtured and nourished into a real and true faith. Those who are visiting must combine spiritual wisdom with psychological understanding for it is only in this way that sound mental health is to be achieved. The spiritual and sacramental ministry of an experienced priest is an invaluable part of the total psychiatric care afforded to those who are mentally afflicted.

The pastoral care of the discharged psychiatric patient, the person who moves out of the enclosed community and enters the larger world, is of vital importance, for often it can be a traumatic crisis especially for a long-term patient. It needs to be understood just what discharge really means to the patient. Both hospital chaplains and parochial clergy should be aware of what is happening, be in touch with one another, and be available to meet existing needs. There may be reactions of fear and insecurity, or dread of rejection by friends in the community. Neighbours and acquaintances may be guarded in their presence and may quite innocently communicate suspicion and distrust.

The former patient should be helped to regain his emotional strength before he is overwhelmed with an abundance of friends and visitors, but there should be no need to 'keep guard' over him, or plan his life for him. He should be encouraged to live as normally as possible, to maintain his self-confidence and to shoulder squarely his responsibilities once more. Those who have spent time, no matter how brief it has been, in a psychiatric hospital or unit experience a sense of shame or stigma, and such feelings are sometimes unfortunately supported by families who are embarrassed by having had a member mentally ill. Embarrassment can all too readily be communicated to the patient who needs the genuine supportive ministry of a caring community which fully understands and openly accepts him. He needs to be nurtured, motivated and guided within an atmosphere of trust and goodwill.

Ideally, ministry to the family should commence early after the admission of the member to hospital. The situation can then be shared with loving care and support, and rehabilitation anticipated in the community with the family, who should be encouraged to ask why the patient behaves in the way he does and what can be done to help him. They must accept the fact that he is sick and appreciate that what he needs most, apart from the obvious psychiatric help, is acceptance, support and understanding. Living with and caring for a mentally ill person can be great strain, and it is necessary for those concerned to use all the tact and forbearance they possess.

It should always be borne in mind that neurosis has a valuable contribution to make to life. 'In a mental hospital', writes Jean Vanier in *Community and Growth* 'it is often the patients who are the most prophetic people ... (p. 191). Every Christian community must realise that not only do the weak need the strong, but also that the strong cannot exist without the weak. The elimination of the weak is the death of fellowship'. (p. 29–30). Mental illness is not a horrible complaint that has seized the person as a chance victim. It has a purpose and a reason, for it is trying to achieve something. Once the neurotic person is aware of this he gains courage to face his personal problem. The love, compassion and understanding of a caring community will begin to open up a way to recovery and growth, and may even be a help to the eventual healing of the patient. Before we attempt to minister we must take a considerable amount of trouble with our own psyche and character, for if we know nothing of our own 'neurosis' we shall merely be projecting it on to others and be trying to correct troubles in them that are really our own. A therapeutic relationship entails a knowledge of ourselves, an honest dealing with our personal fears and anxieties. Healing can only take place when we realise and are willing to accept our own weaknesses and failings. We have to be vulnerable enough to show we really care.

Finally it must be remembered that even some of the more bizarre patterns of the disordered behaviour of the mentally ill can be deeply meaningful. They need to be seen as significant expressions of the inner life of the patient which represent but blind attempts to resolve his various emotional problems and conflicts. The mentally disturbed are letting those around them know they are ill and troubled. It should be readily acknowledged that we have much to learn from them, for it is they who in dramatic and enigmatic yet prophetic ways point us to some of the weaknesses and tensions of our modern contemporary society.

Chapter 8

The Dying

To minister effectively to the dying we have first to be prepared to come to terms with the meaning of our own dying and death, for not until we ourselves have worked out fully the purpose of life and the meaning of death can we hope to be of help and support to those who find themselves in the valley of the shadow of death. No matter how experienced we might be, or how often we have ministered at the bedside of the dying, there is still a sense of awe and uneasiness as the drama of death unfolds itself. It is imperative therefore for the priest to watch closely his personal feelings, for his own anxieties and inhibitions can impede and interfere with his pastoral care unless he has first put his own house in order. It is only then that he will be able to be truly available and sensitively responsive to the various needs of those to whom it is his privilege to minister. No one can give to others a confidence which he does not have himself.

Ideally a relationship should be fostered with the patient before the terminal stage of his illness has been reached. A stranger, be he priest, doctor or social worker, arriving on the scene in the final stages of an illness can be not only disturbing but disrupting to the patient's peace of mind. If the sick person has had opportunity of talking about some of the things which are causing him stress and mental discomfort during the initial period of his illness the priest is then the more able to anticipate some of the fears and anxieties which may arise during the later and more acute stages.

Emphasis should be laid on continuity of care. There may possibly be one person with whom the dying patient may wish to talk and it is extremely important that that individual, be he doctor, priest, nurse, or family member, should not, at any stage, have to withdraw. Better not to become involved at all than subject the patient to the added burden of being deprived of one with whom he is able to relate and in whom he can confide. There can be no substitute for *presence*, for readiness to 'watch and wait', to stay, to be silent in an atmosphere of spontaneous love and care. What matters at the bedside is not 'doing' but 'being', the presence of one who can talk calmly and unemotionally, and who can listen quietly and assuredly. The priest must needs listen skilfully and sympathetically for clues which indicate either a readiness to discuss or a desire to remain silent, for it needs a keen sensitivity to pick up the spoken and non-spoken symbolic language of the patient. Often the patient is not only willing but anxious, at some level or in some way, to share his dying experience with others.

The dying seem to be able to deal with their dying and pending death more effectively and assuredly than those who care for them. It is we ourselves who frequently become threatened and uncomfortable when fears of death are openly expressed and questions about dying freely asked. It is for this very reason that the dying patient finds it difficult to find someone at his bedside who is prepared to stay and listen, to sit and watch with him, giving all they possibly can of their affection, respect and love.

The prospect of death arouses a wide range of emotions which include despair, resentment, anxiety, defiance, help-lessness and fear. A great deal of the fearfulness of impending death has been learned throughout life. If we have not confronted our own dying and death inevitably we shall be shocked and unprepared when it eventually catches up with us. More prominent than the fear of death can be the fear of dying, which may include the fears of pain, the unknown, loneliness, separation from family and friends, loss of identity, self-control, of becoming a burden. Symptoms such as nausea, immobility, incontinence, cause patients much distress and vicariously also those around them. It has already been noted (see p. 25) that in sickness there is often a sense of isolation from oneself and from others. Such loneliness is reinforced by the fact that others tend to avoid a sick person. This mutual withdrawal is even more pronounced when one is dying. The closer to death the more the withdrawal. Visits become less frequent, and duration of time spent with the patient decreases. The impact of all this is a greater sense of isolation and an increasing fear of loneliness. 'The relentless falling off of visitors hurts so much', confessed one dying patient. 'I'm not good company now, so I'm not wanted, and I cannot but feel bitter and childishly resentful. I feel that I need to cling to anybody, like a hurt child. All I ask is a little company, kindness, any indication that I am not forgotten'. Loneliness can be one of the worst of all human experiences and apart from relief of pain probably security and companionship are among the prime needs of the dying. Those who help most are those who give to the patient the feeling that they are with him, and interested in him, thereby diminishing the tendency towards isolation and abandonment. For example those who in effect are saying, 'You matter. You will not be left alone. You don't have to worry that what can be done is not being done. I am with you'.

A certain level of awareness of self and one's body is a necessary precondition to suffering. The fear of pain is not merely a physical fear, but a fear of the unpleasant, and feelings of anonymity and meaninglessness can exacerbate pain. Pain can be physical, mental, social or spiritual, and fortunately much can now be done to alleviate it in its varied forms. Many people believe that pain is inevitable in terminal illness, but modern studies have shown that of those who die of all forms of malignant disease some fifty per cent are unlikely to experience pain at all; ten per cent may be expected to experience mild pain only, and the remaining forty per cent experience severe pain. Analgesics used are now able to alleviate, indeed abolish, pain while the patient himself still remains alert and able to enjoy the life that goes on around him. Much comfort can be given to the patient by explaining that death is usually not a painful affair. This is true for a variety of reasons, frequently because of the nature of the particular illness, partly because many patients lose consciousness or awareness at the end, and also because of the efficiency of medical care. A patient's confidence in the nursing staff, as well as the assurance of a listening ear, of a companion who is prepared to sit alongside him can contribute much to the relief of his pain. Pain is often found to be most intense when the patient is left on his own, and the presence of another does much to comfort and console. If a dying patient knows he is being loved in the true sense much of his distress and discomfort may be relieved. Mental and social pain can often prove more hard to bear than physical pain, and it is the person who has the time and the ability to listen who helps most. Much mental suffering may be caused if a dying patient feels there is no one around to whom he can communicate his hopes and fears for what lies ahead, and he needs to be afforded both time and opportunity to express his fears and to come to terms with himself and his illness.

When the dying are near their death they seem to lose much of their fear and there often seems a willingness to die. Rosemary and Victor Zorza in their book, *A Way to Die*, (Andre Deutsh, 1980), which is an account of the terminal illness of their twenty-five year old daughter, Jane, describe how her main fear was resolved: 'There's only one thing that worries me. I wish I knew what it was going to be like—dying, I mean. I'm a bit scared of that, but I suppose nobody knows. . . .' Julia (one of her hospice nurses) looked at her gravely. 'I think I can tell you', she said. 'You'll just go to sleep and slip away without waking up'. She spoke quietly, but with assurance. There was a moment's silence while Jane absorbed this. 'That sounds good to me'. Julia went on, 'I've watched a lot of people while they died, and that's what will most probably happen to you'. Jane was content. Now free from the constraints of the future, free of possible disciplines that she would resent and probable defeats that might crush her, she had only to deal with the present, and it was manageable, limited, under control. She seemed to have no fear left in her'. (pp. 222–3).

The normal initial reaction when a sick person is brought face to face with the reality of death is to be shocked, to deny, negate, or turn aside. Death happens to other people, not to oneself! Denial is a very common mental mechanism to dispense with a perceived danger, and the dying have a tendency to euphemize their troubles. Denial nullifies part of the reality, and restores a state of previous harmony for a while. It can be a very useful defence for it gives the patient necessary time to become accustomed to the idea until he can cope with the reality. Many a patient will maintain denial until the moment of death while another may not need it after the initial shock. The mechanism of denial can last a few seconds or drag out over months. It may sometimes seem rather a puzzling process for family and friends, and they may feel rather embarrassed and unsure of how to respond, for the process seems to fluctuate from hour to hour, day to day. The dying have a tendency to deny more to some people than to others, according to how they expect each person will respond to what they say. If denial helps the dying patient to face up to life with a greater degree of freedom, then it is helpful and should not be disturbed. Attention must always be paid to what the sick person himself wants and not what others may feel is good for him, and he should not be expected to conform to the ideals or expectations of public convention.

Denial may be accompanied by anger, hostility, or feelings of resentment, directed against anyone, the hospital, the doctor, God, or those who are striving to do their best to help. The existential fear of separation often expresses itself in this way. The patient should be given full and free permission to vent such negative feelings and be assured that they will be met with understanding and support. Anger can be very hard for family or friends, doctors and nurses, to deal with, for it seems impossible to please or to reason. The most helpful way for all concerned is to treat the patient with patience and understanding, and listen such criticisms and complaints out. Such outpourings will relieve the patient's feelings, and there will be no need to agree with everything expressed. Anger and hostility can be positive and thera- peutic functions and do not always have to be repressed or controlled. The moods of patients tend to swing and change almost daily, and often there is emotional confusion. JoAnn Kelley Smith, a dying patient, wrote in her book, '*Free Fall*', (S.P.C.K. 1977), a rather vivid description of such a conflict: 'I'm not sure why, but I want to accept, and I end up rejecting. I want to love but often show hostility. I find peace but am often afraid. I am willing to surrender but more often seek to control : I seek joy and find sadness : and I have a faith but live with insecurity'. (p. 72). If the patient has had the com- panionship and understanding so sorely needed during this period then a stage of calm acceptance may finally be reached. It is important to recognise a distinction between being willing to die and explicitly hoping or wishing to die. Active acceptance is completely different from passive resignation. Acceptance produces something positive and vital to the patient while passive resignation, being essen- tially negative, casts a shadow of gloom across this final phase of the patient's illness.

The vexed question of whether the dying should be told or not has no standard formula ; each patient must be treated as an individual. So often it is the dying who tell us and not the other way round. There are some patients who are strong- minded whilst there are others who are over-sensitive and highly emotional. There will be a number who seem to sense their true condition and its prognosis; some who are prepared to accept the diagnosis but not the prognosis. There are, however, probably far more patients than is sometimes realised who prefer to know the truth. A nagging fear, together with a dwindling hope, is often far harder to bear than the thought of impending death. Fear of the unknown is sometimes more difficult to bear than fear of the known. Whatever information may be imparted to the patient he will eventually find out about his illness in various ways. The real question is how freely should we talk about dying in any particular situation. At this stage communication is all important. 'The question should not be "should we tell . . .?"' writes Dr. Kubler-Ross, 'but rather "how do I share this with my patient?"' (*On Death and Dying*, Tavistock, 1970. p. 32). The patient himself should be the one to take the initiative and he should be allowed to bring up the topic in his own time and in his own way if he so wishes. Truth should never be forced upon any unwilling patient. When he brings his existing feelings out into the open they can be dealt with honestly and openly. To lie is rarely or never justifiable. Far too often in a conspiracy of silence and deceit all sorts of 'games' are played with evasions and untruths. It has been said that 'truth is a vital drug, the only problem is getting the dose right'. It is not so much what is told but how it is told that matters most. If the priest is perceptive and sensitive to the needs of the dying patients to whom he ministers; if he is prepared to watch with them at the bedside and not hasten to retreat, he will be better equipped to gain that insight to understand and appreciate their true feelings and thoughts. He will be ready to help those who wish to express their deepest longings and innermost questionings, and, on the other hand, he will respect the feelings of those who wish to remain silent and not have the true facts disclosed to them. His whole approach will need a great deal of tact, skill and patience. Much emotional relief can be gained from frank talk when the patient and his family are freed from the strain of concealing their own personal feelings—'we can say a lot when there is nothing to hide'. Not every family however is able to discuss such matters openly with the patient and, where this is so, reticence must be accepted and understood. Often the priest will serve as a 'mediator' when the patient himself wishes to be open and explicit with him and yet expresses his inability to speak as freely to his wife or next of kin. He will not of course 'take sides', but, wherever expedient, serve rather as a 'catalyst' to resolve emotional tension or 'blocking', and in this way help to promote a further understanding and acceptance.

Truth does not altogether cancel out hope and the aim of pastoral care will be to provide continuous support for the dying. The hope to be encouraged and fostered will be entirely realistic, prepared to reckon with the worst, and not built upon naive and impractical ideas. It is the little or simple hopes which often need to be encouraged and wherever possible met—'I'm hoping to see my grandchildren tomorrow'. 'I hope to get home for a few hours over the weekend'. 'I hope to watch the TV this evening'. Hope must be retained to the end. As Dr Lammerton once remarked, 'Hope should only die just before the patient'. Patients should never be left to feel that the doctor has played the last card and that 'nothing further can be done'. The caring, the comfort and the love will continue until death itself occurs. The goals and hopes of the dying are very simple and often flexible; for one day or one hour may be all they are able to cope with, yet they can still be full of expectation.

Where should the final days of life be spent—hospital, hospice or home? Such a question has no straightforward answer, for what matters most are dignity, comfort and peace of mind. If such conditions as these can be achieved at home, with the full support of domiciliary services, then surely home is the place in which to die. Over half the deaths in this country occur in hospitals and only a third at home. More than a quarter of hospital bed–days are taken up by people who will be dead within a year. This means that for the majority of people their last days are spent in a clinical and institutionalised setting. With advances in medicine, medical technology and managerial functions, there has been a shift of emphasis in most large institutions. In recent years they have become more and more geared to the objectives of accurate diagnosis and acute therapy, and a greater concentration is laid upon preventive and curative measures. Such advances in technology, exciting as they may be, often make it more difficult for personal and human aspects of nursing to be carried out and time given to the slow pace and simple needs of the dying patient. There seems less and less time in the life of a busy hospital ward for those who need the all important simple comforting care, for the maximum attention is demanded to meet the more urgent and immediate calls of the critically ill. As soon as cure becomes irrelevant care immediately becomes the all-important factor, for the dying patient needs all the nursing skills to enable him to be comfortable and secure in mind and body to the very end. In the clinical and academic atmosphere of a larger hospital there is the ever-present danger of him being seen as 'a failure' for whom nothing further can be done.

With the upsurge of interest in the care of the dying has come the hospice movement. A 'hospice', in mediaeval times, was a resting place where pilgrims were welcomed during their travels. The modern hospice, whose main concern is to tend the dying, can be a wonderful haven of peace for those who are travelling towards the end of their life's journey. There are at present about fifty hospices in Britain and their aim is to work towards 'a good death' with dignity and personal attention, as well as the use of drugs to curb suffering and needless pain. 'Death can never be made easy, but it can be made holy, and that more than anything else is the secret of a hospice'. (*The work of the Hospice*, Sister Paula, Nursing Times, 19 April 1979. p. 667). Studies carried out comparing hospice care with that of the ordinary hospital show that those patients who are nursed in a hospice remain more mobile, suffer less severe pain and anxiety, and their families also show less anxiety and are able to spend more time with the patient and far more time talking to staff, other patients and other visitors. Another advantage is that patients' families are more likely to be able to help care for their patients in a practical way, and also to know the members of the medical and nursing staff personally who are involved in the care of the loved ones. With control of some of the common symptoms of terminal illness and the alleviaton of pain in all its aspects, dying patients are thus enabled to live to their maximum potential.

Many of the hospices are religious foundations, established as charities, and working with the support of the Department of Health and Social Security. Some have teaching centres in which medical and nursing students and members of the caring professions gain experience on ward-rounds, in seminars and discussion groups, thereby playing an important role in present-day medical and nursing education. Other important contributions of such specialised units are that they are small and the standard of nursing care is usually very high, being carried out with a deep sense of vocation and dedication. Patients are accepted just as they are, able to maintain their own individualities, and have all the comforting measures which tell them that they are still important people. Many hospices have home-care programmes to care not only for those not yet admitted but also for other patients who have been discharged temporarily. In such a programme nursing staff work in co-operation with the general practitioners and community and social agencies. Approximately ten per cent of patients are able to go home from hospices for periods of time once their symptoms are controlled. Open days and the valuable service of voluntary workers all help to foster good community involvement.

Terminal care support teams now function in some of the larger teaching hospitals and the domiciliary based support schemes look after the dying at home. As well as the care of the patient such teams also support and teach staff and relatives and help families at the time of bereavement. 'Hospice at home' schemes are being pioneered to offer hospice-style care for people who are terminally ill and those suffering intractable pain from any cause, and they bring this care to patients in their own homes through their home care service.

Given the choice the majority of dying patients would probably choose to die at home, among familiar surroundings, members of their family, and all that has made life dear to them. Home provides stability and familiarity, and death is after all essentially a family affair. Families normally go to very great lengths to care for their loved ones at home, but sadly there is often inadequate provision of services available to help them. On the other hand many seem ignorant of what resources there are to help in their local area. Often relatives themselves are elderly, and more women are out at work, so it becomes difficult to share in the care, support and responsibility of nursing a very sick person in the home. Good and effective services to provide for both patients and their families are most essential, and the community nurse should be aided by the complementary services of health visitors, home-helps, night-sitting services, with the general practitioners at the helm. It is to reduce much of the strain and suffering of the dying and their families that the hospices have extended their scope to provide domiciliary services to nurse patients in their own homes. It is important for the family to be reassured that, should they be no longer able to cope, there will always be a bed available for their patient in the local hospital. In spite of some of these considerable difficulties of home care it is preferable, wherever possible, for the dying to be surrounded by the members of their family and to take their place in the normal activities of home. Here children are able to share in the family's concern, for illness is a family crisis and they should be allowed to help and shown they have a part to play.

Like birth death is a family affair and pastoral care of the dying must also include that of the family. Care of the family is after all part of the care of the patient. An important part of the priest's role will be to help the members of the family come to terms with the patient's inevitable death. This will alleviate much of their pangs of grief and be of much support to them in the various stages of bereavement. Some family members begin to withdraw emotionally from the dying patient because they find the experience too painful, while there are others who wish to draw closer. Often relief is expressed when honest and open communication becomes possible, perhaps after weeks of pretence. Where there is difficulty in relationships the loneliness and isolation of the dying person is accentuated. Often the very ill may manifest aspects of character which are quite out of keeping under normal circumstances and they may appear to be petulant and ungrateful. These traits can cause much distress to the family and it is important to point out to them that these are but common emotional reactions associated with terminal illness, and that they need not feel guilty or blamed in any way.

Some terminally ill patients, overwhelmed, as often they are, with fear and loneliness, wish to discuss spiritual concerns in an endeavour to resolve some of their feelings of isolation and uncertainty. Others seek solace in priestly and pastoral ministrations in order to help them put their affairs, material and spiritual, in order. Many seem to have little or no religious belief and adopt an attitude of an inevitable fiat— 'this is it!' Each attitude has to be respected, and each need met. There will be no place for playing on feelings of guilt; no attempt to erect barriers of communication with pious clichés and ritualistic dogmas or reasonings, for these only serve to threaten and abort any meaningful relationship between priest and patient. As a representative of truth and honesty the priest can give confidence and courage without glossing over the reality of death with superficial and banal reassurances. Through a ministry of sharing and caring, of presence, prayer and sacrament, he can assist the dying patient to live what period of time remains to him with a sense of worth, dignity and meaning. He can help him strive not so much for self-preservation as for self-fulfilment. He can encourage him to gain a truer perspective on life and see that health is not the ultimate end of life. Help may be given to the patient to grope for values that transcend both health and survival and so be ready to surrender himself up to a faith that can encompass even pain, suffering and death itself.

It will be necessary to adopt various methods of approach to meet the particular needs of each individual patient. It is what the priest is at the bedside of the dying that will prove far more effective than what he either does or says. His manner must bring calm and serenity and his whole being bear evidence of one 'who has been with Jesus'. It will be paramount time for listening and entering into the deepest silence with the patient, being responsive to his thoughts and values. Often theology will have to be held in abeyance, and impulsive needs to reassure and smooth things over put aside. Method and technique will be secondary, for the primary concern of the priest will be the extending of a relationship, pointing beyond and beneath himself to God. In touch with the patient he will listen for the question behind the question, for the fear behind the bravado, for the insecurity behind the pretence, and for the faith behind the timidity.

Terminal illness can create a deep sense of disintegration with its accompanying anxiety and insecurity, and physical contact can be of much support. To hold on to an outstretched hand in loneliness and pain provides a sense of attachment, reassurance and comfort. It is a gesture which transcends verbal limitations and human boundaries. It symbolises that whatever may happen the priest will be there, doing all in his power to help. 'You are not alone. I am with you'. Such an assurance cannot be spoken—it has to be lived.

Hearing is the last of the senses to go, so it is expedient to talk to comatose patients as naturally as to those who are conscious. In this way their dignity is still being respected; they are still being seen as persons to be loved and respected. It is advisable to assure the members of the family that the patient can hear, for such assurance gives them hope that there is still a vital communicating link between them. The presence of the priest at the bedside, his being there, will afford a therapy of companionship which will help transform despair into hope and give light in the midst of darkness and futility. To stay with the dying patient, to watch by him, to relate to him, to communicate with him, without necessarily knowing all the answers, is to symbolise our togetherness as a family. Such companionship is a kind of redemptive presence that becomes in itself a healing process.

Groups of caring layfolk can provide a most worthwhile and valuable service to the dying by assuring the members of the family that they are prepared to be available whenever required, no matter what the need, what the hour. When the patient is at home friends and relatives may well be over-tired and worn out with uncertainty, sadness and anxiety. They should be allowed plenty of opportunity to talk and discuss their problems, fears and concerns. Local parishioners may well arrange a rota of members to sit up with the patient by night to relieve the family and allow them some sleep. By day they can make provision for them to go out for a break occasionally. In this way an atmosphere of trust, goodwill and christian fellowship can be fostered. What such a lay ministry can mean is described by the parents of Jane, in their book, *A Way to Die*. 'The promise that Jane wouldn't be left alone was easy to keep. Two old friends . . . sat with her for long periods. Sometimes we talked, sometimes we sat in silence. . . . The presence of these friends were a great comfort to us, helping Jane on her last journey. It was a link with all the bedside vigils of past centuries when relatives and friends silently watched and waited. It was a reminder that death was inevitable, a natural part of life's pattern, not an isolated event that was destroying Jane, but a universal experience' (p. 236). What it means to those who are prepared to undertake this vital lay service to the dying is recorded in a letter to the *Church Times* (Dec. 1979). 'The whole parish supported the family (of the dying) in its prayers . . . for the eight women involved so deeply it was a profound experience, and each one feels that she would never again be afraid to help in a similar situation'. As a learning encounter those who so serve will soon discover a mutuality of ministry. Sitting at the bedsides of patients who are experiencing the peace, tranquillity, and dignity of fulfilment in death, they will have grasped something about the drama of life for themselves. The closer we come to these things the less we shall fear them when our turn comes.

Finally let us always remember that the dying can be our spiritual guides, helping us to get things into true perspective. By ministering to them we shall often learn more than we can teach, and receive more than we can give. Our living can be enhanced by their dying. When heart speaks to heart dying can be time of maturity, growth and spiritual awakening for all concerned, and it will be part of our love and care to help make it so. If death can once again become a family experience shared with caring friends within a community of fellowship and love, then we may well recover many of its lessons and values which are at present sadly being lost in an age of clinically isolated and professionalised dying. 'We, the care-givers are being cared for—unable to help themselves they heal us'.

Chapter 9

The Bereaved

In the care of the bereaved, priest and laity alike are faced with some of the most difficult and profound experiences both emotionally and spiritually. Those who grieve will need understanding and acceptance of their feelings far more than soothing ready-made solutions to their problems. Bereavement, like death, threatens and disturbs, and in our embarrassment we search for quick solutions to complex problems, and are more prone to advise than listen, and to prescribe than counsel. Feelings of inadequacy are accentuated too by the poverty of verbal communication for words in themselves do not seem to be sufficient. Mere expressions of sympathy or feeling sorry for the bereaved are not enough, and to make our ministry meaningful involves a depth of insight and understanding. The counsellor has to understand as fully as possible what this bereavement means to the family members concerned and to be able to communicate such understanding and sensitivity.

There are approximately three million widows and eight hundred thousand widowers in Great Britain. For every six adult women one is a widow; for every eighteen adult men, one is a widower. Recent figures show too that there are two hundred thousand children under the age of sixteen who have lost a parent by death. As well as an ever deepening understanding and appreciation of the christian meaning of life and death those who attempt to comfort and console the bereaved will need also a thorough appreciation of psychological insights into what goes on in the feelings and experience of those who mourn. Unless there is a keen recognition and understanding of those traits much harm will be done by the uninitiated and inexperienced. Where the counsellor, on the other hand, is familiar with some of the basic elements of bereavement and grief, and is calm and confident himself, much strength and support can ensue and even such painful events can be translated into occasions for growth.

Before dealing with some of the more normal reactions to the grief situation attention should be drawn to a rather neglected area of pastoral concern, that of preparing the family for bereavement. Much anticipatory grief work can be accomplished before death actually occurs, for grief really begins at the stage when the next-of-kin are informed that the patient will not recover from his illness. Anticipatory grief, if handled aright, will help in the adjustment of the family at a later stage in the actual bereavement situation. In his ministry to the sick and dying the priest has an unique opportunity to help prepare the family and relatives for the grief processes which are to follow; for where a good working relationship has been established during the terminal illness the way is open for the facing of feelings that begin to find expression, and anger and guilt, when they arise, can be ventilated openly. Should ambivalent feelings exist, they can begin to be released as the death is being anticipated. Now too can be an opportune time to anticipate some of the family's reactions. Are they the sort of people who are highly emotional? What are some of the inter-personal relationships within the family? Are they such that will lead to resentment, jealousies, bitterness? Do they easily panic? Because of his knowledge and perception of the total family picture and his understanding of some of the dynamic factors at work the priest is in a most strategic position to be able to detect any danger signs or trouble spots which can so readily develop when bereavement eventually occurs. No matter how lengthy the terminal illness may prove to be, when death itself takes place its finality will always prove a shock and will release emotions which its anticipation could not. Some will have doubts about the efficacy of prayer; others will have guilt feelings coupled with anger and bitterness. The working through of much of these feelings can often be anticipated and they themselves saved from a great deal of self-reproach and remorse. If some of these features of the grief situation can be explained and understood as natural and normal, the family members will then be prepared to recognise their feelings for what they are.

Bereavement and the grief which follows have no clear-cut bounds; rather are they processes which have to be worked through, the more fully and freely the better. Grief comprises a very complex set of psychological and physical reactions which follow a very similar pattern in the majority of those who are bereaved. These reactions are by no means to be seen as separate stages, neither are they successive or of fixed duration. The bereaved go through them at their own pace and sometimes manifestations of two stages express themselves almost simultaneously.

The first response is generally one of *numbness or shock* which is nature's method of dulling the initial emotional pain. In its more severe manifestations shock generally lasts only a short time. It can take many forms and express itself in a variety of reactions. It does not necessarily occur at once but usually within a few minutes, and it can then last for a few hours to a few days. In some circumstances the bereaved will often seem stunned and remain transfixed in silence, being totally unable to 'take in' what has happened. They seem inconsolable and completely distraught. Others may give full vent to their feelings and become extremely agitated and angry. There will be people who will suffer from delayed shock and face up to things with a cool exterior, but at some later time the real shock strikes them with an added severity. Feelings of emotional distance from other people are common and are graphically described in Susan Hill's novel *In the Springtime of the Year* (Penguin, 1977). When her friends come to offer their condolences to Ruth on the sudden death of her husband, Ben, 'they all seemed to be a great distance away from her, even as they filled up the small room, she heard what they said as though it came from down a long tunnel'. (p. 31) Everybody and everything seem unreal and remote.

Shock may be followed by a period of *disorganisation* in which the bereaved find they are unable to carry out the most ordinary everyday duties. It may also have the opposite effect, for it varies enormously from individual to individual, and some may be able to organise affairs in a most efficient and conscientious way and then totally and suddenly collapse. As with any intense feeling, grief will also produce a number of bodily symptoms. These include loss of appetite, weight, difficulty in sleeping at night, digestive disturbance, palpitations, headaches, and muscular aches and pains. Extreme restlessness and inability to sit still are common.

The next stage, usually transitional, is *fantasy* or *denial*. The bereaved cannot take in the full impact of the situation. Although most common in the early stages of bereavement this defence mechanism may recur throughout the entire grieving process. 'I can't believe it's happened'! 'It can't be true'. 'He'll be back, I know he will', are often the verbal expressions of denial. Often in its milder form it will mean that the bereaved person is prepared to acknowledge the death but cannot quite face up to his feelings. He does not deny the reality of the situation, but he tempers the reality by trying not to acknowledge the full impact of his emotions. There may be 'searching' behaviour which will include waiting for the dead person to come home from work, looking for the deceased in the street. 'I saw my husband walking towards me, but when I got really close I could see that it wasn't him after all', remarked one recently bereaved woman. Sometimes a disconcerting effect of bereavement takes the form of 'hallucinations', of seeing or hearing the dead person. Such hallucinations can be very vivid and the bereaved person may reach out to touch or speak to the loved one who has died. In Charlotte Bronte's *Jane Eyre*,

Mrs Fairfax reflects—'Sometimes I fall asleep when I am sitting alone and fancy things that never happened. It has seemed to me more than once when I have been in a doze that my dear husband . . . has come in and sat down beside me; and that I have heard him call me by my name, Alice, as he used to do'.

As denial breaks down, *depression* often emerges and may last for some time. An aching void has been created within the family circle and a sense of apathy and depression envelops the bereaved. Depression will be coupled with an inability to make decisions, which are often so necessary at such a time. One form depression can take is that of desolate 'pining'. Pining and searching seem to go together, with a persistent wish to look for the person who is gone, a preoccupation with thoughts that can only give pain. This search for 'something to do' is bound to fail because the things the mourner can do are not, in fact, what he wants to do at all. What he really wants is to find the 'lost' person. Despair consequently brings with it feelings of helplessness and hopelessness, a realisation of the powerlessness to bring back the dead person. As time passes, if all goes well, the intensity of pining diminishes and the pain of pining and the pleasure of recollection are experienced as a bitter-sweet mixture of emotion, 'nostalgia'.

The transition between initial shock and the full expression of grief is often complicated by feelings of *guilt and recrimination*. These emotions are directed towards oneself, the deceased, other people and God. A bereaved person may search for evidence of failure in his attitude during the events leading up to the death. 'If only I'd sent for the doctor earlier!' 'Why didn't I realise how ill he was?' Guilt can be both real and imagined, for actual negligence to the deceased or for an angry thought, word or feeling, and often actual and neurotic guilt will merge into the other. Recrimination may also be directed towards the person who has died. 'He's left me just when I needed him most'. 'Why have you done this to me?' The majority of people will probably work through these feelings, but some seem for ever to live in a state of relative adjustment with very little genuine acceptance. A common experience is irritability in respect to other people, with unaccustomed feelings surging to the surface. The individual wants, yet does not want, to be left alone.

Undefined feelings of *anger* and *resentment* are often present—a feeling that people just do not understand. Aggression may be directed against those surrounding the death, doctors, chaplains, nurses, who did not prevent it from occurring. There is a protest against God or fate—'Why did you do this to me?' Anybody or anything that brings home the loss is reacted to as a major threat. Relatives and friends are often surprised and sometimes hurt by the indignant responses of the widow or widower. It is as though in the mind of the bereaved they are obstructing the search for the one who is lost. There are occasions when the bereaved will take death personally, seeing it as something done to them, and so they seek for someone or something to blame. Value judgements may be made, such as older people should die before younger, 'bad' people before the 'good'.

It is only by working through anger, guilt and recrimi-nation that whole-hearted grief can be expressed. Often the individual will have the *urge to weep* and this should always be encouraged without being forced. He should be helped to express as much grief as he feels, no more, no less. Some will immediately give vent to tears, others will be 'like a monumental statue set'. No one should be encouraged to grieve if he feels no grief, but neither should he suppress his emotions in conformity with public convention.

Resolution and acceptance take place in the majority of instances suddenly or gradually over time. The waves of feelings become less and less intense, and the bereaved person begins to go through a period of adjustment, which is a continuing, almost never-ending, yet absolutely necessary process. He begins to control the initial intensity of grief, but it is always there. The work of grief, as C. S. Lewis explains in *A Grief Observed*, is a winding valley, and the mourner will experience repeated feelings of anger, disbelief and recrimination before the reality fully asserts itself and full-fledged therapeutic grief ensues. Pangs of grief can occur, for example, when a photograph may be found in a drawer, or at birthdays, anniversaries, and festive seasons such as Christmas. People naturally differ in the length of time necessary to 'let go' of the dead person and to reorganise their lives, realising that 'life must go on'. Most people need one or two years to recover from a major loss. There is no short-cut or escape from this process of 'working through' grief, as it is a normal natural thing that must take place—indeed *will* take place. It is the price we must pay for love, for being attached to someone. Only by working through the difficulties with christian perspective can the necessary yet painful events be translated into occasions for growth. If the process follows a normal course, as it fortunately does in the majority of instances, the bereaved person can readily adjust to what has been a most shattering experience. Adjustment merges into acceptance, and the bereaved reorganise a life in which the dead person has no place. There will however still continue to be regressions to previous stages, with melancholy and loneliness, and memories or incidents that open the wound once more. In the normal process although the scar remains the wound gradually begins to heal.

After outlining some of the more common symptoms of normal grief it might be helpful to mention briefly some of the signs of abnormal reaction, for in his pastoral care of the bereaved the counsellor should always be alert for 'danger signals'. Of the morbid grief reactions there are two forms— the *delayed reaction* and the *distorted* one. Delayed reactions are often mobilised perhaps years after the bereavement and because of an event which is similar but has no apparent connection with the earlier one. Should another death occur in the family the original emotions may be mobilised, and the grief reaction actually deals with the first bereavement rather than centring on the more recent loss. When the first bereavement occurred there was probably very little grief expressed, and deep misery was concealed under a brave and bold front. In distorted grief reactions there occur agitated depression, suicidal tendencies, feelings of unworthiness and of intolerable guilt. Often there are long periods of severe self-reproach carried to excess, and unless skilfully handled by the counsellor such a long-continued state of depression and melancholia may lead to a marked psychiatric illness or episode. The almost complete withdrawal of the bereaved from society with no inclination at all to take up again former social and interpersonal contacts will be another sign of abnormal grief. There may also be a complete reversal of normal attitudes to everyday life and existence. Self-punitive behaviour becomes marked and all consideration of the future 'thrown overboard'. There is also a group of psychosomatic disorders which are linked with the grief syndrome—ulcerative colitis, asthma and arthritis. Another danger sign is when pastoral care seems of little or no avail and the bereaved continue for months in a static or regressive state with no desire to be helped and with no urge to work through their grief.

It must be emphasised that fortunately the majority of people work through the painful and stressful stages satisfactorily in varying degrees, and where there are signs of abnormality the priest should not shoulder alone the full responsibility of pastoral care. In many instances it will be found that signs and symptoms of emotional disorder were prevalent before the bereavement occurred. Important and serious consequences following bereavement have been found to be frequent. Bodily symptoms may result in substantial ill-health, and emotional distress may develop into well-recognised psychiatric disorder. Studies have shown that of those persons admitted to a psychiatric hospital the number of patients whose illness followed the death of a spouse was six times greater than expected, suggesting that bereavement must have been one causative factor in the development of the illness. Another study has shown that widows under the age of 65 consulted their general practitioner because of psychiatric symptoms three times more frequently than they had done during a control period before the bereavement. It is also recognised that for some time after the death of a spouse, a widow or widower runs a considerably greater risk of dying than married people of the same age. The increase in mortality occurs in the first two years after bereavement and is particularly marked in the first six months, when there is a rise of about forty per cent in the expected mortality rate, the mortality rate for widowers being twice as high as that of widows. A high proportion of the increased death rate after bereavement seems to be due to heart disease, especially coronary thrombosis, which makes the theory of a 'broken heart' a very real phenomenon.

A particularly vulnerable group at risk are bereaved children. Between the ages of three and ten a child tends to pass through three different phases in his ideas about death. The young child, from about three to five, denies death as a regular and final process. To him, death is like sleep; you are dead then you are alive again. Or, like taking a journey; you are gone, then you come back again. For this reason a child of this age may seem very callous to an adult when he is told of the death of a member of the family. He may express an immediate sorrow, and then seem soon to forget all about it. Between five and nine years it has been found that a child tends to personify death, not yet accepting it as a final process. Not until around the age of nine does a child first begin to recognise death as inevitable for all persons, and as something that can come to him. Three main questions seem to arise in a child's mind concerning death. What is death? What makes people die? What happens to people when they die and where do they go? In attempting to answer these questions the age of the child and his concepts of death must be taken into account. The child's first need is not a theory of death but a sustaining affection which becomes a source of reassurance. As in the case of a birth in the family, a child's questions about a death should be answered simply, factually, without evasion, but without the obligation of going further than to answer truthfully the questions that are asked. When there is a chance to prepare the child for an impending death this should be done, for it is always better to prepare than to spare him. The reaction to the loss of mother or father takes a variety of forms, the most common being a mixture of aggressiveness and withdrawal. Guilt clouds the child's inner world and he may see his naughtiness as responsible for his parent's death. Frustrated by some order or chastisement, a youngster might say, 'I hate you', or mother, overtired and fatigued at a child's continual temper tantrums, might so readily exclaim, 'Johnny, you'll be the death of me!' Is he therefore the cause of the tragedy? he asks himself. He may want to punish himself for thinking thus, and may therefore deliberately do things that he knows will cause punishment, which will be his way of working out his guilt feelings. The surviving parent should try to discover the worry and alleviate it. But it is the child who is docile, quieter and more withdrawn than before, who is in danger. His parents may take this as a promising sign and remark with confidence, 'It's wonderful how he's taken it. He never mentions it at all'. Inwardly he may be mourning acutely, and without help can carry the wound of bereavement throughout life.

It is essential for parents to watch for any change of behaviour, however small and insignificant. Above all the bereaved husband or wife should try to show their grief openly and share it with the children. The aim of all those who are helping the bereaved child and his family, for help cannot be given in isolation, must be to prevent the child feeling rejected. Children are normally tough and resilient and if adequate care and support are given they are able to cope with the tragedy of a death of a parent. It is not so much the bereavement in itself but the way in which it is dealt with that affects the future health and happiness of the grief-stricken child. It is important to make sure that it is known what the child has in mind before questions are answered.

There is little point in answering questions that are not being asked. When parents are frank and honest about their grief feelings it makes it possible for their child to feel part of the emotional life of the family, for he will feel much safer and more secure being included than excluded. Honest answers can be handled far more easily than dishonest and deceitful evasions. As death is natural so it can be described to him in natural terms. A bereaved child can stand tears but not treachery, sorrow but not deceit.

There are obviously no clear-cut rules as to what one says at times of bereavement and one will take one's cue from what the person or family appear to want. The priest and those who try to help will avoid offering trite and over-confident advice. There must always be a readiness just to be with those who sorrow. Many really need people to talk to and who will listen to them, and to be able to express exactly how they are feeling. There will be moments when they will want to be alone with their personal thoughts and memories but that should not be an excuse for leaving them alone altogether. The wise counsellor will speak sparingly and listen attentively, gently encouraging the bereaved to talk about the deceased and to express their emotions freely. The sooner they can begin to get out their real feelings and work them through, the sooner they will be able to adjust and accept their new situation. Grief work has three ingredients. There is first of all the acceptance of the loss and of the suffering that accompanies it. Then will come the review of the past shared experiences and activities, in order to realise the full extent of the former relationship. Finally there will be the realisation that each area of life has to be readjusted to function in the absence of the person who has died. Such grief work must come from within and be done by the bereaved themselves. There are no short-cuts to inner growth and maturation and each situation will be different.

It is wise for the priest to be aware of his role and how the bereaved see it. He must try and sense what they expect of him, for in this way he will be able to get some tentative guidelines as to how he is best able to help and support. The problem is set out by Murray Parkes (*Bereavement*, Tavistock Publications, London, 1972). 'Pain is inevitable .. and cannot be avoided. It comes from the awareness of both parties that neither can give the other what he wants. The helper cannot bring back the person who is dead and the bereaved person cannot gratify the helper by feeling helped. No wonder both seem dissatisfied with the encounter'. The counsellor's skills will be evident in his handling of each necessary stage, for he can easily be so emotionally involved that the dangers of an over-sympathetic approach must be avoided and the traits of transference and counter-transference watched. The bereaved person has lost a love object and can so readily transfer affection to someone who offers concern and understanding. If he counsels wisely he will be able to empathise without becoming emotionally entangled, and will avoid all forms of excessive consolation which may inhibit the grief process. Pious and premature interpretations of what the person feels—such remarks as, 'all will be well', 'time will heal', 'I know how you are feeling'—will either go unheeded by a person who is overcome with sorrow or will imply that 'you just don't understand'.

Insight, understanding, compassion and patience are essential needs for those who are attempting to help. There is often a tendency to want those who are grieving to recover quickly, and it is therefore important to keep stating that such feelings are natural and necessary and to show that other people share them. One of the major problems of the bereaved is that of loneliness, and sorrow tends to become more and more painful through being kept secret. Unfortunately so often the bereaved find themselves cut off from those around them. Their friends become embarrassed, not knowing quite what to say to them, and seem unable to communicate with them as ordinary human beings. 'You find out who your real friends are', the bereaved say, meaning that there are certain people whom they have known very well who are just not able to come and visit them any more. What a challenge here for every congregation, for carefully selected visitors who are sensitive to other people's needs. A few who have experienced bereavement themselves and worked through it can assist immeasurably. Because of their courage the bereaved can take courage too. Fortunate indeed are they who can say, 'Yes, I have very good neighbours and friends'. So easily can the bereaved become a threat, as it were, to the local community, and to its emotional stability. Contemporary society's inability to accept the reality of death and its corporate denial of any real help to the bereaved tends to produce an ever increasing number of casualties. Man evades the issue of his mortality. How relevant is the cry of Job when in the very heart of sorrow and despair he exclaims, 'My brothers stand aloof from me, and my relations take care to avoid me. My kindred and friends have all gone away, and the guests in my house have forgotten me'. (Job 19. 13, 14).

There is a great need for a caring and on-going ministry throughout the post-funeral stage. Regular visits should be paid and meaningful relationships built up with the family and its members. The death of one member of the community should be the concern of all. The caring community will use its initiative and imagination to arrange a constant touch with bereaved families by ringing them up, or preferably calling in to check if they are managing all right. Let them be invited out for a meal, and included in social invitations even if they do not feel like coming alone. Friends will provide a ready ear when needed, a shoulder to cry on and a sensitivity to know what to do and when.

The utmost discretion needs to be exercised however, for attempts to push the bereaved into the responsibilities of group participation before they are ready for them may only frustrate and discourage them to the extent that they will further withdraw. Letters of consolation are much ap-preciated, and those who are bereaved will often speak with great gratitude of the number of letters they have received, and the tokens of respect of their loved ones, as if they somehow shared the esteem represented by them. Such messages of condolence must be one heart speaking to another rather than an occasion for explanations. 'Ex cathedra' statements are poor substitutes for those which spring 'ex cardia'. Letters should look at the situation realistically; hard words not to be avoided or coated over with euphemisms, and an endeavour made to leave a clear opening for further correspondence.

There comes a stage when the bereaved person stands in need of reassurance that his sorrow and grief have now sincerely shown his love for the deceased and that the time has come for reconciliation. When such an approach is handled discreetly a turning-point can then be reached. This phase is vividly described by C. S. Lewis. 'Something quite unexpected has happened. It came this morning early . . . my heart was lighter than it has been for many weeks . . . suddenly at the very moment when so far I mourned her (his wife) least, I remembered her best. It was as if the lifting of the sorrow removed a barrier'. (*A Grief Observed*).

Bereavement is the sharpest challenge to our trust in God and many who grieve often look around them in vain for certainty and conviction of belief. The faith of the church through prayer and sacrament, and the love, care and concern of its individual members, should always be available to sustain and strengthen those who can accept it. Those who do not possess a personal faith can nevertheless be consoled and comforted by the understanding and compassion of those around them, even if they themselves cannot believe it. The priest and his people by their friendship and concern can help guide many of the bereaved to a greater capacity for drawing on the love of God, and to discover anew that the experience of bereavement can bring the eternal world very near and prove itself stronger than death.

Voluntary organisations who help with the bereaved include

the following:—

    Cruse, Cruse House, 126 Sheen Road, Richmond, Surrey.

    The Society of Compassionate Friends, 50 Woodways, Watford, Herts.

    The Camden Bereavement Project, 25–31 Tavistock Place, London, WC1.

    The Foundation for the
      Study of Infant Death, 5th Floor, 4 Grosvenor Place, London, SW1.

    Gingerbread, 9 Poland Street, London, W1V 3DG.

Chapter 10

The Various Resources

All healing is from God and as such is an aspect of the present redemptive activity of God in the world. Health is not simply the absence of something wrong such as disease or pain, but the presence of something right. It is soundness rather than physical prowess, of body, mind and spirit. Healing should therefore be seen not as an isolated static event but rather as a dynamic process. 'I have come that men may have life, and may have it in all its fullness'. (John 10. 10). Wholeness is often compatible with physical weakness, for life is valued more for its quality than its longevity. Indeed if used aright disabilities can become instruments of healing. Symptoms may be alleviated, disease eradicated, functions restored, yet to be truly healed the spiritual side of man's nature has to be taken into account and an endeavour made to serve God with heart, mind and strength. No matter how sound physical, mental and social aspects might be, without the spiritual the total picture of man is less than complete. Sadly far more seems to be known about how to combat sickness than how to promote and further health, which has a far wider and deeper connotation than is normally given to the term in everyday speech. Too often it is narrowed down and confined solely to the physical and the mental. The doctor in Camus' novel *The Plague* did just this. Both he and the priest had been deeply moved by the death of a young child by the plague, and Paneloux, the priest, sits down beside Rieux, the doctor, conscious that in their attempt to help those who were suffering they were working side by side for something that united them. 'Yes, yes', says Paneloux, 'you, too, are working for man's salvation'. Rieux tries to smile. 'Salvation's much too big a word for me. I don't aim so high. I'm concerned with man's health; and for me his health comes first'. Rieux was forgetting that salvation means health. To heal is to 'make whole', for health, wholeness and holiness all have a common derivation, and restoration of physical and mental faculties must always be seen in the wider context of salvation.

The Report of the Archbishops' commission on *The Church's Ministry of Healing* (CIO, 1958) stated that 'those who are called to minister to the sick have the duty of setting free all of God's resources for health. They must contend with *all* that interferes with the process of healing. Since certain of these factors, such as anxiety or fear, are on the emotional or spiritual plane, many sick people are in need of assistance which medical science by itself cannot supply ... the pastoral and sacramental ministry of the church ... helps to break down barriers deep in the personality which stand in the way of healing ... by evoking the response of faith it allows the divine grace to act creatively and so determines the issue for health in ways beyond our present scientific methods of measurement'. In illness and disease it is the entire person who is sick. In healing therefore it is the entire person, body, mind and spirit which must be ministered to.

'God's resources for health' derive from the gospel itself and among them are prayer, counselling, penitence, holy communion, the laying on of hands and holy unction. Both psychological and sacramental approaches are inseparably joined together and should work in complete harmony with medical and surgical methods of healing, for the sick need the best that both church and medicine can bring them. It should be emphasised too that these resources make sense only if practised and developed not in isolation from but in complete harmony with all that is taking place in the caring and loving community. The local church and its congregation must be involved in the health needs of the community as well as in the work of the local hospital and sick rooms of the parish. Health always implies a community.

The church lays upon all the duty to *pray for the sick*; at the sacrament of holy communion . . . 'we commend to your fatherly goodness all who are anxious or distressed in mind or body; comfort them and relieve them in their need; give them patience in their sufferings, and bring good out of their troubles'. (Rite A: ASB 1980); 'Save and comfort those who suffer, that they may hold to thee through good and ill, and trust in thy unfailing love'. (Rite B: ASB 1980); in the Litany . . . 'heal the sick in body and mind' (ASB 1980), and in Morning and Evening Prayer when bidden to ask those things which are requisite and necessary, as well for the body as the soul. (BCP 1662). The teaching of the church is founded on the bible and Christ's own ministry to the sick. 'Is one of you ill? He should send for the elders of the congregation to pray over him . . .' (James 5.13). To intercede for the sick means that as members of the body of Christ the priest and his people bring to the feet of Christ the needs of their fellow-members, for 'God has combined the various parts of the body . . . so that there might be no sense of division. . . . but that all its organs might feel the same concern for one another. If one organ suffers, they all suffer together'. (1 Cor. 12. 24–26). If there is a sick person in hospital or at home he should therefore be the concern of all members of the congregation. Through their prayers, through their faith, they will co-operate with all the ordinary means of healing that God has given. What an enormous support it is to the sick to know that they are being continually remembered in prayer through the intercessions of the worshipping community, and that in their weakness they can lean heavily on the prayer support of others within the body of Christ. What fellowship can be fostered when members learn how Christ meets the needs of sick people, and to see with the four friends in the gospel story (Mark 2.1f) how sin can be worse than disease; that effective intercession means resigning sick people into God's hands unreservedly in complete love and trust, not demanding nor dictating, not pleading nor persuading, but bringing them to the feet of Christ and leaving them there in perfect confidence and expectancy. 'John, Betty, David . . . these whom you love are sick'. In interceding for the needs of the sick there will be no need to give medical details, for these are apt to raise doubts and reservations in the minds of some who find themselves dwelling more on sickness than health, more on the problem than the person. Those who pray should feel perfectly free to express hopes and desires for the sick, telling God they want to see them as he himself wants them to be. They will be prepared to allow their whole selves to be engaged in their intercessions and be ready for their thoughts and expect-ations to be purified and brought into obedience to the will of God. It is the congregation which is the healing body and all intercessions for the sick will be linked with those of the people of God, in the context of the whole church, the community of intercessors, of which the prayer-group is but part. It is to this 'best way of all' that St. Paul directs his readers in 1 Corinthians 13, where the on-going work of the congregation in its corporate loving and caring ministry is seen as the real healing power of his body, the church.

A dynamic answer to the question of when to pray at the bedside, in sick-room at home or in hospital ward, centres in the needs of the person who is sick. The priest or the visitor will pray or not pray according to the need of the patient for prayer. He must listen to the person in crisis for leads which will indicate that a ministry of prayer will be appreciated. He will follow those leads by asking the question, 'would you like me to pray with you'? An effort must always be made to sense the sick person's need and to respond to it. There should never be any firm rules or regulations such as *always* or *never* to say a prayer, for 'there is no law dealing with such things as these'. (Galatians 5. 2). One of the difficulties of the 'pray always' concept of prayer is the motive. It should be asked, whose need is being met? Does the priest pray because he needs to, or because the sick person needs it? Those who minister must be open and receptive not only to the promptings of the Holy Spirit but also alert to the spiritual state of the patient. Short extempore prayers at the bedside can often lift up the special needs of the patient in a way that a set prayer may fail, in that it lacks direction and purpose. Sometimes it may be sufficient merely to let the sick person know that he is being remembered by name at the eucharist, in the prayer-group, or to assure him of one's own personal prayers. On occasions it may be more expedient to suggest that a period of silence be kept so that each may pray as he wishes. Often the patient himself will ask for a prayer to be said, and when this is so, prayers should be short, simple and direct, natural, informal and unobtrusive. Whatever the circumstances prayer at the bedside should never be forced nor artificially introduced.

Praying with the sick should be costly. By our stripes they are being healed. If our prayers are to mean anything to God they should mean something to ourselves. Prayer and care should always go hand in hand. The whole congregation is linked together in the family of God, and it is only as prayer-life and everyday life interpenetrate, and love for God and man blend, that they become true intercessors of the sick. As well as *saying* their intercessions they will also be *doing* them. Prayer is no substitute for action. 'I am, often, I believe, praying for others when I should be doing things for them', confessed C. S. Lewis. 'It's so much easier to pray for a bore than to go and see him'! In some way or other those who pray for the sick must also be prepared to share their pain and suffering. 'Here I am, send me'! (Isaiah 6. 9). Only if they are prepared for this to be so can they be truthfully fellow-workers with Christ, for the cost of intercessory prayer is their share in the cost of redemption.

The patient, dependent on his physical and mental state,

can be shown how best he himself can pray in his sickness by just being himself and talking to God, telling him exactly how he is feeling, without necessarily confining his petitions to so-called 'spiritual matters', but merely expressing his desires in his own way as naturally and simply as he is able. Sickness can often be a wonderful opportunity for one has time to pray, to get to know God better and become more and more aware of his presence. For one who is sick the simpler and shorter his prayers are the better, and he will be helped to pray as he can and in whatever way he can. Prayers in sickness can very easily and readily become self-centred and subjective. One way of remedying this defect will be to commence prayer with God before thoughts are centred on self, for then there will be more praise and less petition.

In prayer the sick may be led to try to unite their sufferings with those of the crucified Christ, offering themselves and their sufferings, feeble and weak instruments though they be, as channels through which his works of redemption might be wrought. As they speak to one to whom 'all hearts are open, all desires known, and no secrets hid', they should be helped to realise that they need never be afraid to take to him their anger, resentment, or whatever bitterness they may sometimes feel in their depression or despondency. They can be reminded that much of their loneliness or seeming isolation in prayer might possibly be overcome when they realise they never pray alone but always against the background of the praying of the whole body of Christ, as corporate members of his church.

It is often helpful to teach the sick the use of 'affirmations', short yet strong expressions of faith, which they can use at any time, particularly in periods of great fear or anxiety. Ejaculatory or 'arrow-head' prayers can also be the means of casting out depression or despair by interspersing thoughts of God throughout the day. They will prove particularly beneficial when under temptation, in pain, or when lying awake at night. Jeremy Taylor in his *Holy Living* (chapter iv) mentions how an ejaculatory prayer can be used 'more or less, longer or shorter, solemnly or without solemnity, privately or publicly, as we can or are permitted . . . for we may pray in bed, everywhere and at all times, and in all circumstances and it is well if we do so'. When the physical condition of the patient permits it, his sickness can be an opportunity for praying for others. Bringing healing to others can be part of his own healing, for prayer is limitless in its expansion, and lengthens its cords as it strengthens its stakes. Intercessory prayers in sickness can become very real, for those who are in 'any way afflicted or distressed' know from personal experience what suffering really entails.

Another 'spiritual resource' in sickness is *bible-reading*. In most hospitals Gideon bibles are available for patients' use. If the sick are too weak to read for themselves they can be read to, should they so desire it, by those who visit them. There are now many and various revised editions of the scriptures and there may be certain preferences expressed. The elderly will probably still treasure the familiar language of the authorised version, while younger patients may derive more satisfaction and comfort from the latest versions. If read slowly and reverently the scriptures will reveal the very words of Christ, the very deeds of Christ and the very looks of Christ, and speak to each specific situation. It may be helpful to concentrate first on the gospel narratives, reading short portions, thinking of their deeper meanings and turning them over and over in their minds, so that the very Christ himself, speaking, healing, dying, rising, will make his presence real. As well as the gospels, the psalms too are full of healing and comforting words. One of the main characteristics of the psalms is their naturalness and their relatedness to the whole of life—its doubts, fears, problems, sorrows, joy and delights. As well as deriving consolation from scriptural readings the sick may find much help and inspiration in works of poetry, biography, memoirs, treasuries of devotion and anthologies.

Devotional literature, when used, should be the language of well known and well loved words, for familiarity gives strength. The print should be large and clear enough for tired and weary eyes to read and pain-filled minds to ponder. Short words more often than not are the strong and meaningful ones in our language and have a special appeal to those who are sick. Such literature should be chosen to speak to the needs of the patient and it is most important that it be theologically sound. Some leaflets and pamphlets pander to the emotional and sentimental, and create quite unrealistic expectations and raise false hopes. Devotional literature should always be seen as a guide to a deeper spiritual life rather than a key to solve problems or smooth over difficulties. It should also contain thoughts and truths that will stand up to repeated and continual usage to enable those who are sick to 'read, mark, learn and inwardly digest'.

Pastoral counselling of the sick is another essential part of the total task of the christian community and needs a thorough understanding of the psychological, emotional and spiritual needs of the individual patient. To help sick people may often seem to be a slow and time-consuming task, and indeed it is only right and proper that it be so, but it is the primary charge laid upon every member of the church. If the priest is knowledgeable about some of the ways in which people become anxious and depressed; if he is alert to the many opportunities before him in sick rooms at home and in hospital, then together with members of his congregation to support and sustain him and those who are being helped, much can be done for the mental and spiritual health of those committed to his charge. Together they will be concerned, albeit in a limited way, to help people to be themselves. The warmth of their bearing in the presence of the sick, the sincerity of their intention and the depth of their spirituality are traits that cannot be manufactured by methods or techniques, for they are perceived in ways other than the spoken word, the kind deed or 'a bedside manner'. It is these and not the methods which make the christian counsellor. Counselling entails a measure of that sympathy which means literally suffering with the person concerned.

It must be recognised that pastoral counselling is something far more profound than the giving of advice or information; its emphasis lies in self-understanding and insight by the counsellor rather than the sick person being told what to do. Much experience and skill are needed for it is not an easy task to assist people to grow. The key concept will be *relationship*, a relationship of empathy with a deep sense of identification. It is the love of our neighbour which Simone Weil once described as 'creative attention'. It is the love that every parishioner has the right to expect from a fellow parishioner. When this love is offered with openness and honesty, in the service of acceptance and understanding, it works as leaven, a leaven which lightens and dissipates the burden of suffering and brings renewal of integrity and health in its fullest sense.

Fear, resentment and indulgence along with other negative forces can play no small part in the level of personal health, and a sick person may need to make a formal or informal *act of confession*. Penance will also form a necessary preparation and background for the healing sacraments of holy communion and holy unction. There may be practical difficulties about hearing the confession of a sick person who is among other patients in a busy hospital ward. It is probably somewhat easier however to have some noise going on rather than the whole ward to be held in an artifical and enforced silence. If the patient is ambulant he can be taken along either to the hospital chapel or to a nearby side-room of the ward. With the very sick and weak patient it will not always be possible for a formal act of confession to be made, and in such circumstances the priest will use his discretion and be aware of the place of vicarious faith, penitence, and conditional absolution. There will be some patients who wish to make a general act of confession, and here the priest will assure them of God's mercy and forgiveness should there be true and sincere repentance on their part. In his ministry to the mentally ill the priest must be careful to distinguish the pathological sense of guilt which arises from psychological trouble, from a real sense of guilt. Absolution, coupled with spiritual counsel, can be of much help to the emotionally disturbed patient who is brooding over particular acts of sin, or to the physically sick person who, for example, realises how some besetting sin is sapping his spiritual prowess, and might possibly have played a part in the causation of his illness. Absolution is granted by the authority of the priest who will be acting not only for God but also on behalf of the fellowship of the church to which all belong. Jesus refused in his healing work to concentrate solely on the ills of the body. When a paralytic was brought to him on a mattress bed (Mark 2.1) he was able to diagnose the real trouble which underlay the outward manifestation of it which was the physical paralysis. He saw that if there was to be a complete and permanent cure the whole man must be dealt with. First his relationship to God and to his fellows must be put right, then his physical healing would follow and there would go back to his house a man every whit whole.

The sacrament of *holy communion* gives to the sick grace to withstand the power of evil and enables them to grow into the measure of the stature of the fullness of Christ. Apart from the healing aspect of the sacrament, it is the church's supreme act of thanksgiving and intercession. At the bedside the priest will normally use an abbreviated form of the service, for the elements will have been already consecrated in the parish church or hospital chapel at a previous celebration of the eucharist. It is helpful if the shortened form is printed on a card or leaflet so that patients are able to follow the content of the service without undue strain or stress. Frequently it is found that owing to the difficulty of administering the chalice to those who have to lie flat and still in bed, it is helpful either to dip the host into the wine in the pyx and place it directly into the patient's mouth, or to administer a host previously intincted with wine at an earlier celebration of the eucharist. The printed card should include suitable prayers of preparation and thanksgiving and be given to the patient the evening prior to the reception of the sacrament, for the more preparation taken the more the sacrament will mean to the sick person. The communicant patient should always have something definite to pray for, some substance for confession, some item of thanksgiving to offer, and a definite resolution to make at the service.

The essential ingredients of preparation will be faith in the mercy and goodness of God, repentance and a firm intention to live in charity with all. The thanksgiving will include gratitude to Christ for his coming to serve and feed the sick, and for his presence with them and in them, as well as in all who will be ministering to their needs. The recipient will try to discover some small practical token of gratitude which can be offered throughout the day, expressing thanks not only with his lips but in his life. He can picture Christ at the last supper or on the cross, recall the glory of the resurrection, and his promise, 'Lo I am with you always'. He can be led to think about some of the sayings of Jesus: 'I am the bread of life' (John 6. 35); 'This is my body: this is my blood' (Matthew 26. 26); and 'He was made known to them in the breaking of bread' (Luke 24. 35). Dependent upon their circumstances the sick can thank God for all their many blessings received and for all that is at present being done for them. They can tell God quite simply what they have done wrong and ask for forgiveness for the ways in which they have failed him. Finally they can pray for all those they love, for other sick people, for all in need, and for themselves that their sickness may bring them closer to Christ and his healing power.

In the sacrament of holy communion many a sick person will find direction and purpose for much of the seeming meaninglessness and futility of his illness, faith for the fear which constantly torments him and reconciliation for the estrangement he commonly experiences in hospital ward or sick room. Unfortunately when the sacrament is administered in a hospital ward there is often no one else present apart from the priest and patient. Here is a wonderful opportunity for a few members of the local prayer-group or of the ward staff, as representing the community, to be present, supporting priest and patient and enabling the sick person to look for his healing from the wholeness of the whole body. Here in action is the life of the kingdom, kindled by a eucharistic and sacrificial readiness for living in community, for when patients share together the body and blood in a hospital ward they are expressing their fellowship with one another in Christ Jesus. A sense of nearness, a consciousness of relationship with him becomes so real and vivid that they are turned away from all else to him, and so lose fear of loneliness or isolation.

The laying on of hands is a sacramental act which can be administered either formally or informally. The priest, together with representatives of the worshipping community, may lay hands gently but firmly on the sick person's head. With priest and people participating, the laying on of hands becomes a corporate act. As hands are laid on the head of the patient there will be a period of silence, followed by a short prayer. The hands of the priest will be representing those of the whole church laid on the sick in sympathy and compassion, the congregation thereby showing its concern, demonstrating its love and symbolising its commitment as a caring and healing community. In this sacramental act the sick are able to offer up themselves and all their needs to God in complete trust and absolute confidence, with a ready acceptance of God's will whatever it may be. Physical recovery, although very naturally in the minds of those who are sick, will not be the prime concern, for healing and wholeness imply something far deeper than the mere relief or removal of bodily symptoms. The imposition of hands is primarily a blessing conveying peace and confidence to the sick person, and when administered there often ensues a deep sense of peace, calmness and confidence.

Anointing with oil in the sacrament of *holy unction*, with its background both in the New Testament and in church tradition, is a symbol of the grace of God for the strengthening of the body and soul in sickness. In Old Testament times oil was used to hallow and to consecrate for the anointing of kings, prophets and high priests. It is seen therefore not only as a sacrament of healing but also one of hallowing. Fortunately in recent times it has been restored to its proper place and usage, after a long period of both misuse and neglect, when it was treated as a last rite for the dying with little or no thought of healing, and being administered 'in extremis' came to be associated with death rather than healing. Holy unction has now gained official recognition within the church at large and has been given canonical authority (Canon B27) by the Church of England. In the Roman Catholic Church, as a result of the Second Vatican Council, it is now no longer referred to by that church as 'extreme unction' but rather as 'the sacrament of the sick'.

The outward and visible sign of this healing sacrament is the anointing of the sick person on the forehead with oil in the sign of the cross, together with the prayer of faith and healing. The oil used is ordinary pure olive-oil which has been blessed either by the bishop on Maundy Thursday, or by the priest himself prior to or as part of the service itself. The oil is used as a symbol, and its definite feel on the forehead can inspire confidence and strengthen faith. The benefits of the sacrament include the hallowing of the spirit, the quieting of the mind, and the allaying of fear and anxiety, all of which may open the way for bodily improvement. Such peace of mind enables the sick to face up to their illness, pain or suffering, with renewed strength and inner calm. This sacrament is normally restricted to baptised members of the church, who understand and use the sacramental life, and it is administered more sparingly than the act of laying on of hands. It is a sacrament generally reserved for those who are seriously ill (but by no means necessarily dying), sick persons in pain, patients facing crisis situations and those whose state seems to be deteriorating. Children as well as adults may be anointed.

The priest will prepare the sick person for the administration of the sacrament by instilling faith, repentance, hope, and supporting him with the prayers of the local congregation, continually upholding those in whose care the patient is and on whose skill he depends. There should be an attitude of complete trust and confidence in a loving God, and a conformity to the will of God regardless of the ultimate outcome of the sickness. Preferably holy unction should be administered within the context of holy communion, before the eucharistic blessing and after the reception of the sacrament. Should the patient be at the point of death the procedure is normally reversed for it is more appropriate to receive holy communion last of all as 'viaticum'.

First and foremost the sacrament of holy unction is focused on the setting, quieting and strengthening of the spirit by the increase of faith in God, trusting in him and submitting to his will. After receiving the anointing the sick person will need to relax and express thanks. Subsequent pastoral care is essential and members of the local congregation may visit the sick one afterwards by arrangement with their parish priest, and so help to sustain the hope and strengthen the faith of their fellow-parishioner. Sometimes where there follows recovery and healing of body, mind or spirit, the patient should be encouraged as part of his thanksgiving to offer his renewed strength for more effective service to God and his church. Often a wonderful sense of peace and joy will be granted to the sick person, without perhaps any significant physical improvement in his condition, enabling him to offer his pain and weakness in union with the redemptive work of Christ, and to be obedient to the mystery of God's will. On other occasions healing may come gradually or in some indirect way. There will be instances when complete healing comes only by means of a happy, contented and dignified death. Of one thing the sick may at all times be certain. The sacrament of holy unction brings a deep sense of peace and tranquillity, assuring the sufferer that 'in spite of all, overwhelming victory is ours through him who loved us'. (Romans 8. 37).

Prayer and sacrament, important as they are in sickness,

will not be complete in themselves without the personal and practical involvement of a loving and *caring community*. The church's ministry of healing is far more comprehensive than official forms of laying on of hands and holy unction. People as well as priest, pew as well as pulpit, are all involved and should see themselves as partners in the mission of the church, working alongside others in the total care of the sick as primary agents of healing. Prayer, counselling and sacrament should be seen as a supplement to, rather than a substitute for, personal action. The time a patient now spends in a hospital ward is becoming shorter and shorter. Consequently the ministry of healing is moving out of the hospital environment into the community. Health and healing should therefore be taken as one of the prime concerns of the work and witness of every local congregation if they are to meet this exciting yet exacting challenge. When the community as part of the living church, the body of Christ, is seen in action, loving, healing, redeeming and sanctifying, a new vitality and power is found, a spirituality attained, and a wholeness discovered to confront the strains and stresses of life. The pastoral care of the sick must be seen as far more the total ministry of the whole church and far less the special ministry of the hospital chaplain or individual parish priest. The local congregation in its caring and loving role must be providing wholesome conditions in which those who were sick are enabled to regain physical strength, mental stability and spiritual serenity.

Chapter 11

The Training

Sick visiting is very demanding, physically, emotionally and spiritually, and those who undertake it will need strict and prolonged training. All who minister must be masters of their craft, and they will need not only pastoral skill but also intellectual insight, especially in the area of understanding human nature and how people respond to sickness and ill-health. Basic questions will need to be considered. What are the major elements of human personality? What makes for emotional and spiritual health? What is health or wholeness? How does psychic conflict relate to physical illness? Such questions will be discussed in relationship to such basic christian doctrines as God, man, sin, salvation, forgiveness. In the study of understanding people the next objective will be how best they can be helped. The priest and his people will seek to use this understanding in ways that will contribute to the spiritual health of those who are committed to their care. They will learn how religion, the church and its people, can function constructively in the lives of those who are in need; how they themselves can play a part in both the prevention and pastoral care of physical, mental and spiritual illness.

Training schemes will of course vary according to local circumstances and community needs; whether the priest is just an occasional sick visitor, or an officially appointed part or whole-time hospital chaplain. *Seminars* might profitably be held at regular intervals either in the hospital or in the community. Ideally these should be both ecumenical and inter-disciplinary, with a hospital chaplain, local general practitioner, social worker, health visitor or any official representative of the hospital and community services present. Speakers can be invited to open discussions on specialised topics relating to different aspects of pastoral care and the ministry of healing. A prescribed book might be studied together, chapter by chapter, in house-groups or training centres. As well as understanding people (including themselves) and the community resources those who minister to the sick should also have some 'know-how'. Practical aspects of ministry therefore, while not the primary objective of training, will be given due attention. The work of counselling will be an essential study, together with the most important principles to follow and some of the common errors to be avoided. In unstructured seminars those present may bring out ideas or material they wish to discuss in problems of counselling in home or in hospital ward. Opportunity may also be given to work through some of the theological implications of the church's ministry to the sick, and to consider together some of the many complicated issues involved in present day medico-moral problems. Some of these training groups or seminars might be formal and planned, while others informal and spontaneous. Their major objective would be teaching rather than therapy, together with a sound basis of knowledge, insight and understanding imparted to those present.

An important aspect of a series of seminars might well be to afford opportunity for those present to become familiar with other professional people dealing with people in crisis, and to understand their approach to mutual problems and concerns. Much can be learnt from the insights and methods of social workers, doctors, administrators, group workers and others. To achieve these ends seminars and groups can be planned with them, in order to understand their role in the hospital and/or the community and the insights and methods used to fulfil their role.[1]

[1] For a suggested outline of weekly seminars arranged over a period of three sessions throughout a year, see Appendix I.

Another helpful method of training is that of *role-playing*, which can be defined as the acting out of real or imaginary situations involving relationship between two or more persons. As a way of teaching role-playing has a number of distinct advantages. The procedure gives the individual an opportunity not only to hear about theories of counselling and ministering to those in need but also to observe some of the dynamics of a counselling situation. Through observing and participating in role-playing would-be counsellors develop a greater sensitivity toward the emotions of other people and gain an insight into some of the problems people in sickness present. Role-playing teaches people the important skill of putting themselves in the place of others in order to understand why the other person reacts as he does in a particular situation. If the group is taking turns at playing the role of 'visitor' or 'visited', each member will take full advantage of the opportunity to observe what the participants will do and so learn to eliminate errors from their own performance. Above all this method of training has the sound virtue of getting people to learn by doing.

There are however a number of things the supervisor or group leader needs to watch for when role-playing is used as part of training. To play a role in front of other members of a group can prove for some people a rather threatening experience. It is wise therefore for the group leader at the beginning of a session to select members who are secure and confident personalities. Seeing others in action in this way will help to encourage other members of the group to take part later. Another precaution is to make sure that those who participate in these training sessions do not confuse role-playing with acting. It is by no means a test of acting skills or abilities, and the participant should not worry unduly as to whether he played his part correctly or not.

It is important that all members of the group be made to participate, and encouraged to make observations. Much of the value of role-playing depends upon the discussion after the official session is over. Such discussion will of course be dependent upon the observations the group makes. This method of training may seem artificial but when conducted by an experienced leader it develops a surprising amount of reality, and at times it becomes just as real as a pastoral call in either hospital or home. If facilities are available 'visits' to the sick can be video-taped in a studio, and played back and discussed with the group afterwards. This affords the added advantage of being able to see oneself at the bedside and to take note of mannerisms, intonation of voice, eye to eye contact, and other important features which can either make or mar a pastoral visit. It also enables the visitor to feel something of the relationship which comes to exist in the give and take of a sick-visit.

A helpful adjunct to training will be the keeping of *careful records* of pastoral visits. Such information, to be kept strictly confidential, has a number of important values. Note-writing provides a record of sick visits which enables those who minister to the sick to examine their understanding and care of the patient. Skill in visiting depends upon an understanding which directs and controls the pastoral call. How does the patient feel? Is he anxious, lonely, bored? What are his moods, attitudes, his interpretation of his illness? What needs are being expressed? Note-writing will reveal whether the sick-visitor has let himself and his own prejudices, fears and apprehensions get in the way, and how far the needs of the patient have been met and been satisfied. The written report will also check the extent of self-understanding and reveal its limitations. The keeping of records will prove to be a clarifying and developing process and serve as a method of self-criticism and self-revelation as well as opening the way for self-improvement. It trains the ability of the priest and his people to recall the most significant features of their bedside visit, the underlying elements which would otherwise be quickly overlooked and forgotten, and it reveals why it was found difficult to establish a relationship with a certain type of patient for example, or why no progress seemed to have been made during the visit.

A written record stands as an assessment of sick-visiting. It will be found extremely valuable to glance at the notes before a second or successive visit is made to home or hospital. In this way the memory of the previous visit is recalled, as well as the visitor's grasp of his thought and need. Written records encourage the visitor to think systematically about his relationships with patients and to plan his approach to them. They also provide a means of learning from one's mistakes and failings and so provide a further opportunity to think realistically about alternate ways of pastoral behaviour.

The records detailing the pastoral call will contain any preliminary data which has been made available, such as patient's name, age, religion, ward, home address, condition. The purpose or plans for the call may be listed—for example, what do I anticipate might be the needs of this sick person? How do I plan to meet these needs? What are some of the specific things for which to be alert, or avoid? There might then follow a short summary of what took place during the bedside call. Listed will be the patient's insights into the meaning of illness to him, his attitude towards illness, family, medical staff. His religious background and resources will be carefully noted—how active in church life? Is he a communicant? Has he lapsed? Has he no christian allegiance at all? What are his immediate spiritual needs? An essential item will deal with the self-evaluation, self-insight—how did I perform as priest, sick-visitor, counsellor, understanding friend? What did the visit teach me about myself? Finally there should be recorded the relationships established with others in the hospital or at the home—did I consult with physician, psychiatrist, nurse, social worker, family, hospital chaplain? Was I helpful to them? What needs to be done in this instance? Difficult problems? Plans for follow-up? The actual experience of note-writing quite apart from helping creative thought, relieves emotion just as it does to tell some understanding listener of problems one is facing. Without such written work there can be no check on one's work. The records will be kept strictly for one's own personal and private use, and should not be passed on to successors lest they be misused or misunderstood.

The keeping of careful records will prepare the way for another exercise which should be an essential part of training—the writing up of *verbatim reports* of pastoral calls. This may well prove an irksome task initially but these reports, if described honestly and conscientiously, will prove of infinite value and provide much pastoral material for open group discussions. As with other written material patients' names are to be kept strictly confidential, and can be referred to merely as 'Mr A' or 'Mrs B'. What is worth saying is worth writing, and verbatim reports written up immediately after a pastoral call when impressions are still vivid and fresh will enable the student to penetrate through the more superficial aspects of some of his bedside calls, and as a result the deeper meanings of his relationships with patients will become more clear and defined. Such verbatim reports will also serve as a mirror of the student's own emotional involvement with those whom he visits. He will gain a further and fuller awareness of his feelings and failings in his relationships with other people, for real involvement is an essential part of any effective and meaningful bedside ministry. Not only will he begin to understand the patient more significantly but also himself more thoroughly.

As with general note-writing, verbatim reports should also commence with any *preliminary data* to hand, any information the priest may have about the person to be visited, such as name, age, church affiliation, or other significant points which afford clues as to pastoral opportunities and spiritual needs. After the initial visit this opening section can be omitted and new information reported under the heading of *additional data*. Next will come an outline of his *plans* for the bedside call. Keeping in mind his function as hospital chaplain, parish priest, or lay visitor, he will outline his preparations and plans for the spiritual care he hopes to bring to the patient. Knowing what he does about the sick person, he will try to imagine the situation in which he will find himself on his visit. He will let these plans help him focus his attention on the person of the patient, and these should be written up and recorded before the sick call. Afterwards he may have to revise his plans, or indeed abandon them entirely. There will then come *impressions* under which will be described his reactions to what he saw in the sick room—a snapshot of the scene of action. He will detail what seemed to be the reaction of the patient on whom he was calling. The actual *pastoral call*, vividly and realistically portrayed will follow, and this will be as verbatim as possible, written as direct discourse. Pauses in the conversation, interruptions, facial expressions will be reported, along with any other clues which may reveal the relationship between himself and the patient. He will write up the actual words spoken and describe his actions as well as those of the sick person's. A *summary* of the pastoral visit will follow, and be listed under three sub-headings—analysis, self-criticism, and pastoral opportunities. The *analysis* will include the priest's own interpretation of the visit, its subject matter, and relationships. Tentative explanations will be offered of any puzzling elements of the sick call, or any inability to do so will be indicated in the report. Present insights will be expounded and pertinent phrases from notes quoted. The visit itself will then be *criticised* from an objective a viewpoint as possible. For example, did it begin satisfactorily? Were there any distracting elements in the situation? Was anything accomplished? How was the sick call concluded? Were the methods used helpful? If the visit was unhelpful what might have been the reason? Under *pastoral opportunities* will be stated some of the more obvious of such openings—what are considered to be the spiritual needs of the individual patient? An attempt will be made to outline the personality resources, the situation resources and the spiritual resources of the sick person.

The final section, which will be *plans for next visit*, will outline what suggestions are thought helpful for the return bedside call. Specific things which the sick visitor is hoping to accomplish may be listed, together with notes as to how best they can be achieved. Some of the things to be avoided will also be recorded. The verbatim report will then conclude with asking such questions as:— What was the most important thing the patient gained from this visit? What was the most important thing I gained from this visit? What were the most important questions as a result of this visit?

One of the disadvantages of the written verbatim report as a teaching instrument is that its value depends completely upon the memory of the student, but if written up honestly and frankly it can become a mirror of his pastoral relationship with the patient. In the report he reveals his own personal attitudes, philosophy, and theology through the responses he makes during the bedside call. The very writing of the 'verbatim' will force him to relive the pastoral visit, and as he comes to a deeper understanding of his own participation in the bedside conversation the insight will lead to a clearer awareness of his own identity as a priest or lay-visitor. When the report is discussed with a supervisor or experienced hospital chaplain or parish priest in the training group, healthy and constructive criticism will arise as the working through of the written material progresses stage by stage. The supervisor should never criticise a student's response to a patient unless he offers an alternative. For example, he might suggest, 'instead of saying what you did at this particular stage, would it not have been more helpful to have said . . .' It will be emphasised that there is no one right or perfect response to the exclusion of all others, and such an assertion will discourage the student from becoming defensive in his replies. What is looked for is a response appropriate to the emotional content being revealed.

The dynamics of the pastoral conversation at the bedside will be discussed to help the student examine his pastoral skills and performance, and thereby improve his competence as a sick visitor. Questions will be raised with group members—why did you break off in your conversation when the patient was about to express her real feelings and doubts?

Could your questions have been worded and framed more effectively to draw out some of the depression and anxiety the sick person was so obviously experiencing? Was there too great a tendency to moralise, generalise, sermonise? Why did you do all the talking? So the discussion may continue with further concerns and questionings being examined and explored. If such criticism can be accepted in a healthy way, without those who participate feeling threatened in the presence of others, such an exercise will prove a learning process in itself and make for further growth and maturity of all concerned. When questionings, doubts, hopes and aspirations are honestly faced and openly talked through, such a ministry of sharing becomes a ministry of learning, and frank discussion will help the student to become more and more articulate regarding his own plan of action and goals.

Hospital chaplains will have much to contribute to the total care of the sick by communicating with other staff members what is going on when they are visiting patients. Such communication may well take the form of a written *pastoral consultation report*, which will be similar to the doctor's medical report, and the social worker's case report. This may well be an extension of the verbatim within the medical consultation model. The entire ward staff will be given a wider view of the patient by chaplains' reports of this kind, which might well be included in the official kardex and form part of the patient's case-history. A hospital chaplain will have impressions of how many a patient feels toward his disease and the treatment processes, and his frequent pastoral calls at the bedside may well help to identify some of the patient's needs which were previously unknown. Not only will such inter-communication establish good inter-personal relationships between chaplain and medical staff but it will also place the chaplain himself in a continual on-going learning experience. Similar arrangements might well be made between parish priests and local general practitioners and members of the community team concerning home visits to the sick.

Those who wish to study pastoral care of the sick in depth should be encouraged to participate in full-time *residential clinical training programmes* in the large teaching hospitals and medical centres. The advantages of the hospital based programme are that sick persons can be seen more frequently than in the community and so more contacts can be made in the same amount of time. Personal supervision of training in a hospital is easier, and the priest-student soon discovers he is not the only professional worker who can help people. He soon realises too that he needs to co-operate with doctors, nurses, social workers and all others who come to bring their various skills to the person in need. In this way he learns not only to work with representatives of these other professions but also to utilise community resources which may lead to more effective living. Training of this kind cannot be adequately taught in classroom or study where theory, excellent and essential as it may be, is not experienced in concrete interpersonal situations. The heart of the clinical experience is the personal encounter with the sick person, and the sharing of this relationship with trained chaplains or parish priests, who have had considerable experience in the field of pastoral care, as well as with his fellow-students who are sharing similar situations and concerns. Such a training programme of three months duration, or of a succession of 'quarters', is a supervised experience which will provide students with opportunities for intensive clinical study of problems in the sphere of interpersonal relationships, and will seek to make clear the resources, methods and meanings of the christian faith as they are expressed through pastoral care.[1] Religious faith and practice have an unique contribution to make toward physical, mental and spiritual health, and such a contribution can be explored and developed in clinical training schemes of this nature and duration.

In-service training programmes might be useful for those who might possibly find a full-time residential course

[1] For suggested programme outline see Appendix 2

impractical. These programmes may be arranged for one day a week throughout a period of months, and would include individual supervision and presentation of verbatim reports, along with lectures, seminars, and supervised visiting. Seminars might profitably concentrate on the ministry of healing, pastoral problems and concerns, ethical problems, pastoral conversation, sacramental ministry, pastoral counselling. Education activities may be arranged in the community so that there is a continuity of pastoral care from hospital to home.

Without adequate training and supervised experience the priest in his pastoral approach to sick people can so easily become irrelevant to their needs. Unless he understands what is involved in his relationships with others, particularly those who make him feel anxious, threatened, or insecure, he will spend a great deal of his time defending and protecting himself rather than helping and supporting others. Those who visit the sick must become aware of their weaknesses and deficiencies as well as their strengths and capabilities, so that they may rectify the former and develop the latter.

As well as the essentials of intellectual insight and the acquisition of pastoral skills the spiritual health of the sick visitor himself will be of paramount importance. What he is will be far more important than what he knows or what he does at the bedside. He cannot really know or do anything rightly unless he himself is right. From the initial question of 'what must I *do* to be of help to sick people?' the sick visitor has to work through 'what must I know?' and 'what must I say?' until he finally reaches the all vital question of 'what must I *be* to be of real help?' This last question will constantly remind the priest that in the face of all the help he may gain from training procedures and programmes, he must never lose sight of his distinctive role as a priest. He is first and foremost a spiritual counsellor, and his spiritual maturity will therefore be of prime importance. It is not so much what he does *for* people, nor yet what he does *to* people, but what he *is* to people that matters most. At a time when pressures and needs of the everyday world appear to multiply, never is it more urgent than now for both priest and people to realise that it is possible to 'labour in vain', to 'spend all night and take nothing'. In I Kings 20.40. are warning words—'As thy servant was busy here and there, he was gone'. The watchword of the pastoral ministry must be *multum non multa*, and no array of statistics to be tabulated in visiting lists can compensate for the lack of 'the one thing needful'— the growth and development of the personal spiritual life. There can be no finer tribute paid to priest or layman if those in sick beds in hospital or at home can say of him what the woman whose house was on the wall could say of the prophet (2 Kings 4.9. NEB) 'I know that this man who comes here regularly is a holy man of God'.

Appendix 1

A Suggested Outline of Lay Training for Sick Visiting

Course outline of lectures and seminars

TERM 1

 1 Introducing the course
 2 The sick visitor and his/her role
 3 Techniques of pastoral counselling
 4 Principle of a counselling relationship
 5 Dynamics of the pastoral conversation
 6 Conducting a hospital/home visit
 7 Practical guidelines for visiting the sick
 8 Writing verbatim reports and keeping records
 9 Pastoral theology and pastoral care
10 Understanding human behaviour

TERM 2

11 The crisis of illness and hospitalisation
12 The crisis of dying
13 The crisis of grief
14 The crisis of guilt
15 The hospital/home environment and routine
16 The role of the hospital chaplain/parish priest
17 Ministering to relatives
18 Worship and the sacraments in hospital
19 The use of prayer
20 The ministry of healing

TERM 3

21 Ministering to medical and surgical patients
22 Ministering to paediatric and maternity patients
23 Ministering to coronary care and intensive care patients
24 Ministering to neuro-surgical patients
25 Ministering to renal dialysis and cancer patients

Appendix 2

A suggested outline plan for a three months' residential clinical training programme

1 *Introduction/Orientation:*
Group building exercises
Expectations of course
Sociology of health care
The health team
Future developments in health care

2 *Counselling:* Both theory and practice, using:
Cases
Simulation
Video
Real world

3 *Role:*
Role theory
Perceived by chaplains
Expectations of patients and staff (tape recordings)
Analysis of difference

4 *Cultural Differences:*
The socio/economic/religious differences of other races
Other faiths

5 *Community Support:*
What components? e.g. Social workers
                    General practitioners
Functions?   Health visitors
                    Community nurses
How to mobilise?   Voluntary organisations
                    Relatives
                    Neighbours
                    Church congregations
                    Church organisations

6 *Ethical Problems:*
Abortion
Sterilisation
Resuscitation
Transplants
Confidentiality
Purpose: Information/Education
         Attitude exchange
         Difficulty of judgemental roles
         Individual counselling

7 *Sociology and Psychology of Illness:*
Sick Role
Stigma
Psychosomatic illness
Psychology of Pain—Thresholds
                  Attitudes
                  Projection
Psychology of care/self help
Institutionalisation
Aggression—victim behaviour (simulation) reasons for aggression
Control of others' aggression

8 *Theology of Suffering and Pain:*
Sin and sickness
Evil and a God of love
Salvation
Psychology of pain
Theology of suffering

9 *Worship:*
Location—Structure
         Chapels
         Wards
         Dual purpose buildings
  Form—Ceremonial
         Interdenominational
         Broadcasting

Patient/Staff involvement in administration and worship
Chapel furniture
Composition of congregation—sermon content/style
Religious continuity in community
Practical problems/issues

10 *Ministry of Healing:*
What is healing?
Healing and wholeness
Prayer and sacrament
Caring community
Health

11 *Care of Dying:*
Terminal illness
Personal attitudes
Where to die—hospital/hospice/home?
To tell or not to tell?
Does the patient know?
Staff attitudes—nursing the dying child
                identifying with patient
Family reaction
Chaplains' ministry

12 *Care of Bereaved:*
Grief—Psychological
       Physical
       Normal vs abnormal reaction
Loss— Practical—House
                Finance
                Social
     Spiritual
Caring organisations
Funerals—Interment/Cremation
        Funeral directors

Experimental learning methods to be used throughout the course.
Close counselling support is a major requirement of course members.
The emphasis throughout the training is on patient care.

Appendix 3

A Typical Ward Timetable in a General Hospital

6.00 am–6.30 am	Patients woken up with cup of tea.
6.30 am–8.00 am	Taking of temperatures, pulse and respiration rates.
	Getting up to wash, or be washed.
	Preparation of patients for operations.
	Sanitary round.
	Giving of medicine, special drugs; performance of special treatments; treatment of pressure areas to prevent bed sores, etc.; provision of mouth washes etc.
7.30 am–8.00 am	Night nursing staff off duty, day nursing staff on.
8.00 am–12 noon	Breakfast
	Provision of medicines; dressings, etc.
	Ward Sister's round.
	Bathing and making beds.
	Newsagent brings daily papers; delivery of letters, etc.
	Visits by doctors, chaplains.
	Mid-morning drink.
	Some patients to operating-theatre, X-ray department, etc.
	Visits from other hospital staff such as medical social workers, physiotherapists, laboratory technicians, occupational therapists, dieticians, etc.
12 noon–1.30 pm	Lunch.
	Handwash bowls; medicine round.
1.30 pm–2.30 pm	Rest period if possible.
2.30 pm–3.30 pm	Further visits by doctors, chaplains and staff (as above).
3.30 pm	Tea.

4.00 pm–6.00 p.m.	Handwashing bowls.
	Beds tidied.
	Taking of temperatures, etc.; giving of medicines, special drugs and treatments.
6.00 pm–7.00 pm	Supper.
7.00 pm–8.00 pm	Visitors.
8.00 pm–10.00 pm	Treatment of pressure areas, etc.
	Hot drinks.
	Taking of temperatures, etc.
9.00 pm–9.30 pm	Night nurses on duty.
	Sanitary round.
	Giving of drugs, sedatives, treatments.
10.30 pm approx.	Lights lowered.

Appendix 4

Useful Addresses

Healing Ministry

Institute of Religion and Medicine, St Marylebone Parish Church, Marylebone Road, London NW1 5LT

Churches' Council for Health and Healing, St Marylebone Parish Church Vestry, Marylebone Road, London NW1 5LT

The Guild of St Raphael, Marylebone Parish Church, Marylebone Road, London NW1 5LT

The Guild of Health, Edward Wilson House, 26 Queen Anne Street, London W1M 9LB

Counselling

The Westminster Pastoral Foundation, 23 Kensington Square, London W8 5HN

Association of Pastoral Care and Counselling, St John's Church, Waterloo Road, London SE1

Hospital Chaplaincy Ministry

Hospital Chaplaincies Council of General Synod, Church House, Dean's Yard, Westminster, London SW1 3NZ

Hospital Chaplaincy Board of Free Church Federal Council, Free Church Federal Council, 27 Tavistock Square, London WC1H 9HH

Church of England Hospital Chaplains' Fellowship, Highcroft Hospital, Erdington, Birmingham B23 6AX

Free Church Hospital Chaplains' Fellowship, Free Church Federal Council, 27 Tavistock Square, London WC1H 9HH

Social Services

National Council of Social Service, 26 Bedford Square, London WC1

The British Association of Social Workers, 16 Kent Street, Birmingham B5 6RD
Association of Community Health Councils for England and Wales, 362 Euston Road, London NW 3BL

Voluntary Organisations
The British Red Cross Society, 9 Grosvenor Crescent, London SW1X 7EJ
Women's Royal Voluntary Service, 17 Old Park Lane, London
The Samaritans, 17 Uxbridge Road, Slough, Berks SL1 1SN

Care of the Elderly
Age Concern, Bernard Sunley House, 60 Pitcairn Road, Mitcham, Surrey CR4 3LL
Help the Aged, 32 Dover Street, London W1A 2AP

Care of the Mentally Ill
MIND—National Association for Mental Health, 22 Harley Street, London W1N 2ED
The Richmond Fellowship, 8 Addison Road, London W14 9DL

Care of the Dying
The Marie Curie Memorial Foundation, 124 Sloane Street, London SW1X 9BP
St Christopher's Hospice, 51–53 Lawrie Park Road, London SE26 6DZ
St Joseph's Hospice (The MacMillan Service), Mare Street, London E8 4SA
National Society for Cancer Relief, Michael Sobell House, 30 Dorset Square, London NW1 6QL

Care of the Bereaved
Cruse Clubs, Cruse House, 126 Sheen Road, Richmond, Surrey
The Society of Compassionate Friends, Secretary—Mrs Brenda Trimmer, 2 Norden Road, Blandford, Dorset

Appendix 5

Select Bibliography

The Pastoral Nature of the Ministry, Frank Wright (SCM, 1980)

The Christian Healing Ministry, Morris Maddocks (SPCK, 1981)

Reaching Out, Henri J. M. Nouwen (Collins, 1980)

The Wounded Healer, Henri J. M. Nouwen (Image Books, Doubleday & Co., 1979)

The Healer's Art, Eric J. Cassell (Penquin Books, 1978)

Watch with the Sick, Norman Autton (SPCK, 1976)

The Patient as Person, Paul Ramsey (New Haven & London, Yale University, 1975)

Community, Church and Healing, R. A. Lambourne (Darton, Longman and Todd, 1973)

Healing and Christianity, Morton T. Kelsey (SCM, 1973)

Basic Types of Pastoral Counselling, Howard J. Clinebell Jr. (Abingdon Nashville, 1966)

The Faith of the Counsellors, P. Halmos (Constable, 1965)

The Pastor as Counsellor, Andre Godin (Gill & Son, 1965)

The Casework Relationship, Felix P. Biestek (Allen & Unwin, 1961)

Principles of Pastoral Counselling, R. S. Lee (SPCK, 1969)

Introduction to Pastoral Counselling, Kathleen Heasman (Constable, 1969)

You Alone Care, Heather McKenzie (SPCK, 1980)

A Private Battle, Cornelius Ryan (New English Library, 1979)

This Bed my Centre, Ellen Newton (Virago, 1980)

Watching for Wings, Roger Grainger (Darton, Longman & Todd, 1979)

Community and Growth, Jean Vanier (Darton, Longman & Todd, 1979)

The View in Winter, Ronald Blythe (Allen Lane, 1979)

The Hospice Movement, Sandol Stoddard (Jonathan Cape, 1979)

A Way to Die, Rosemary and Victor Zorza (Andre Deutsch, 1980)

Free Fall, JoAnn Kelley Smith (SPCK, 1977)

On Death and Dying, Kubler Ross (Tavistock Publications, 1970)

On Dying Well, Church Information Office (1975)

The Dying Patient, Ed. R. Raven (Pitman Medical, 1976)

Peace at the Last, Norman Autton (SPCK, 1978)

A Death in the Family, Jean Richardson (Lion Publication, 1979)

A Time to Die, William Purcell (Mowbray, 1978)

Death and the Family, Lily Pincus (Faber & Faber, 1976)

A Grief Observed, C. S. Lewis (Faber & Faber, 1971)

Bereavement, Murray Parkes (Tavistock Publications, 1972)

The Pain that Heals, Martin Israel (Hodder & Stoughton, 1981)

Rediscovering Pastoral Care, Alastair V. Campbell (Darton, Longman & Todd, 1981)

The Way of the Heart, Henri J. M. Nouwen (Darton, Longman and Todd, 1981)

General Index

Index of Persons

Index of Organisations

Index of Scriptural References